UNLOCKING THE SECRETS OF CANCER

A GUIDE TO CANCER CAUSATION AND HEALING WITHOUT CONVENTIONAL THERAPY

By

James L Andrew

Disclaimer

This information is not intended as a substitute for professional medical advice, emergency treatment or formal first-aid training. Do not use this information to diagnose or develop a treatment plan for a health problem or disease without consulting a qualified health care provider. If you are in a life-threatening or an emergency medical situation, seek medical assistance immediately.

Furthermore, the information contained in this book is the expressed opinion of the author based on their own experience and research dealing with cancer and the medical profession and is not to be considered as medical advice or treatment of any kind, but as educational material only.

Any references to historical events, real people, or real places are the expressed opinion of the author.

First printing edition 2021

theageofignorance2021@gmail.com

Contents

PART V

PART VI

INTRODUCTION

Three things killed my father, fortune cookie advice, primitive treatment, and good old-fashioned ignorance! It's not difficult to imagine the shock someone must go through when they are told they have cancer especially the way society thinks of this terrible disease. The conventional treatment of cancer is essentially assisted suicide that medical professionals get away with simply because the law says so. In medical terms, the treatment of any disease is to only manage symptoms, not cure, and this is why your oncologist will never offer you a solution to your problem beyond surgery, chemotherapy and radiation. Even if they knew of a natural treatment for cancer that carried no side effects and worked they still couldn't give it to you simply because they have not been trained to do so. Doctors who do will in all probability lose their medical licence, be fined and probably go to jail. Today, many people don't realise that this is a reality that many doctors are forced to face as they watch their patients slowly deteriorate. The medical community is divided when it comes to the treatment of diseases like cancer and the scope of how we approach modern disease is severely limited for political and legal reasons, not medical ones.

According to the Cancer Council Australia before the age of 85 1 in 2 men and women will be diagnosed with cancer, what they don't tell you is that approximately 2.1% are likely to live beyond 5 years from their original diagnosis. Cancer has now become the world's fastest-growing disease and according to the World Health Organization between 2008 and 2030 cancer incidence in low to medium income families will have grown by 80% and by

2030 the death toll will exceed 13 million people every single year, far worse than the COVID 19 pandemic.

Cancer doesn't discriminate against cultural or religious beliefs, age, race or gender and can be a formidable obstacle to overcome. It takes its toll on the patient and the people who care about them physically, mentally and emotionally, cancer will test you in ways you cannot imagine, especially if you have chosen to listen to your oncologist and pursue conventional treatment. The future looks bleak for the cancer patient, subjected to brutal and aggressive treatments with low success rates and the ever-present thought of death on their mind, the clock is ticking and little can be done to remedy this terrible disease, or so we are led to believe.

My name is James Andrew and this book is about a spiritual awakening that is growing amongst people who no longer have faith in the system that we have been told to trust and claims that it's there to protect us. This book is about seeing the world in a different light and enlightening people on some of the lies that we have been told to believe and how they impact us everyday.

My journey into the subject of cancer is about a 5-year struggle with doctors, family and friends and how all of these people believed the lies to what has ultimately led to a generation of people who can no longer distinguish the difference between fact and fiction. The lie's we have been told on diseases like cancer are so convincing that they start from the food we eat to the things that we have been told to trust on the supermarket shelf. From sunscreens to weed killers, produce to meat products, even what comes out of your tap at home.

All of these things are contributing to the degradation of your health and professionals like your doctor are asleep at the wheel as to how it is contributing to the increase of chronic diseases they are seeing in their practices. When patients are diagnosed with these chronic illnesses it is simpled explained away by blaming stress or genetics because they have no real answer.

To understand what happened and how this relates to you, you first need to understand what my family was like, like most families we reacted the same way most people would if you had been told you are dying, because in most people's minds that's exactly what they think when they are told they have cancer. At the time we were all ignorant about what was happening and what was going to happen when my father was told he had non-small cell lung cancer which is the most common type of lung cancer you can get. Like most people, my parents were brainwashed by the system into thinking that cancer is a death sentence when in reality it is not, it's a wakeup call! They were the type of people who believed the rubbish on the news every night at 6 o'clock, or on the radio going to work, not to mention all the superficial and unimportant crap that gets published in newspapers and magazines. In my opinion, the only thing the newspaper gets right consistently is the date! For example, front cover news on Kristen Stewart cheating on Robert Patterson, as opposed to page 20 which reads in a tiny article that no one ever looks at called "Fluoride, poison in our drinking water". Even something more recent like Johnson and Johnson's baby powder causes cervical cancer which appeared in The Guardian, where 22 women claimed their talcum powder gave them cervical cancer and that J&J lied to its customers for 40 years about how it was contaminated with asbestos.

You'd think this would be all over the news and in the papers considering how popular this product is, but no doubt a lot of money has been spent to hush it all up especially when the court-ordered J&J to pay $4.7 billion in damages. Its articles like these that give people a false perception of reality and what matters to us as human beings, think about it, even if Kristen Stewart did cheat on Robert Patterson then aside from Robert Patterson would you really give a shit? More importantly, it's their business what goes on like any other couple, so why would the TV and the newspapers care more about 2 people and their little love triangle as opposed to millions of people like Johnson and Johnson's customers and the products they sell?

Anyone who knows me knows that I have never been one to follow the herd and society treats such people poorly, labelling them with titles like a conspiracy theorist, crackpot, dooms dayer, anti-establishment, freak, fake, pseudoscience, quack and hate monger. To someone like me, this is hilarious because all I did was get off my ass and report on what scientists have been saying all along, that is real journalism. I have learned over the years that some people cannot be helped and others have exactly what they deserve coming to them, a universal karma so to speak. These kinds of people are everywhere and in every occupation, and I have never had much time for those who criticise others with their invalid opinions based on nothing, especially when they do nothing to understand them. This is the definition of a die-hard idiot, and you cannot educate an idiot, after all, they will drag you down to their level and then beat you with experience.

The trouble today is that there appears to be a lot of effort directed towards keeping people in a constant state of distraction and obliviousness. When the Roman empire was on the verge of collapse they used the same tactic to keep the public calm because the authorities knew that the public was a force to be reckoned with and they would not be able to control its citizens if they learned the truth of what was about to happen. They called it drink and circus, which is why getting drunk and watching the Gladiators was such a big thing during this time, today we call it alcohol and football with a generous dose of reality TV. People are so conditioned in their beliefs that no matter how logical or relevant you make an argument against what doctors say it is met with skepticism and resistance. This only adds to the problem because their minds are not open enough to accept the possibility that maybe their doctor is just as ignorant about treating their disease as they are.

I have always found conspiracies a subject of intrigue, not to be confused with conspiracy theories, a distinction rarely made by the media when they are trying to humiliate someone who is not in line with their views, like Peter Evans from My Kitchen Rules. However, to truly understand what is going on and how to make an informed opinion you must hear both sides of the argument which is why I always found an interest in cryptozoological documentaries on Bigfoot, Loch Ness, UFO's and the mysteries of ancient civilizations which continues to fascinate. Today, having an alternative point of view gets you labelled as a conspiracy theorist which of course is ridiculous in a democratic society. The reason I mention this is because you must become fascinated and curious about your cancer, this will help cultivate the right mindset and keep your mind open to learning new things, even if those things challenge your world view. We have become so cut off from other possibilities that putting blind faith into everyday things is so common that it screams out how complacent we have become. For example, what do you think the moon really is? Most would say it's a giant rock in orbit around the earth that controls the tides, and on the surface that's a pretty accurate statement. But wait until you take a few more things into account. First of all the diameter of the moon is 3,474km to the meter! and it is approximately 400 moon sizes away from the earth, these are the exact measurements you would need for us on Earth to get a perfect solar eclipse and the chance of this happening by natural processes are so ridiculously small that the implications are even more fascinating. Also, during the Apollo missions, NASA astronauts placed seismic devices on the moon's surface to see what the internal structure of the moon was like, then they crash-landed the Apollo 12 module with an S-IVB rocket which had the equivalent force of approximately 12 tons of TNT and when detonated, in NASA's own words the moon "rang like a bell" sometimes for hours at a time, indicating that it is hollow. Another thing to take into account is why the Earths gravitational pull hasn't sucked the moon out of its orbit and pulled it into the earth? Also, ancient myths from tribes like the Zulu's talk about a time on Earth when the moon wasn't even here and that it was brought here by the God's. Finally, the dark side of the moon has never been seen, so who knows what is really going on there? Ancient aliens did an episode which covered this and other anomalies, but the point I'm making is that even though no one can say for 100% certainty what the moon really is, it's obvious to anyone who bothers to look that it is anything other than just a rock in space.

Those who raise public awareness on controversial matters no matter how unbelievable they sound are those who I have always had a great admiration and respect for, putting everything on the line in the face of ridicule and scrutiny because they dared to question. These people are persecuted by the public when it was them they were doing it for, just to snap them out of this psychotic daydream we call life and teach us to wake up to the things we have been conditioned to ignore. You don't write a book challenging the current paradigm on anything let alone cancer in hopes of seeking fame and fortune, especially when you're telling the truth in a world built on lies. When truth-tellers tell it how it is people often feel as if they are being judged or looked down on by another and this raises a wall that is extremely difficult to lower unless that person is open to change, which sadly, many are not. So this book is for those who possess an open mind and have had that crazy feeling that something is out of place in this world. There is a vital piece of knowledge that has been forgotten over the last 200 years and that is food is not food, food is medicine. In the old days, food and medicine were one and the same, so why is food as medicine condemned in the 21st century? Today these industries have been segmented and are among the largest in our world. In 2014 for the first time, the pharmaceutical industry made more than 1 trillion dollars and is now the most powerful industry in the world.

I would strongly argue that it is your doctor's job and responsibility to give you options, so if alternative treatments can have the same or greater effect than conventional treatment without the harmful side effects then that is what your doctor should be doing. When you start talking about nutrition being the cause and solution to the medical problems that plague us in the 21st century you'll find that in all of their training nutrition is not even a subject of interest because it contradicts the primary education of most doctors, which is to diagnose conditions and prescribe medications.

Like most of us coming up in the world doctors are trained not educated, and yes there is a difference, Mark Twain said that he never let schooling get in the way of his education, doctors are told what to think and not how to think, which these days appears to be a common dilemma in all academia. To reinforce my point you don't have to believe me, just ask your doctor what nutritional training they have had and see what they say. They will probably tell you little if any, in my research over the years I have found that the partners of doctors probably know more about nutrition than they do, which is exactly why many doctors will never recommend anything natural as a treatment to any type of cancer or any chronic illness. There are huge contradictions in the advice you get from doctors and many wouldn't tell you that medical professionals like your GP and oncologist are torn between doing what's right and what is easy. For example, they say nutrition is important and we hear things like "you should eat foods like broccoli which is an anti-cancer food", but after you have been diagnosed suddenly anti-cancer foods like broccoli don't work? This is a huge contradiction in logic and they simply cannot have it both ways.

In this book, you will discover that the advice given to you by your oncologist is generally scripted as they believe in a one size fits all approach. Few would agree that a person's cancer may be as individual as you are, but if you take into consideration what we eat, drink, breath, use on our bodies and our overall habits it doesn't sound so farfetched as no two people use or do the exact same thing every single day. Doesn't it strike you as odd that our approach to cancer has remained the same despite all of our technological achievement? It's a bold statement for someone with no medical certificates to criticize the medical profession about medical issues, but I possess something far more valuable than a piece of paper that says what I can and cannot do, what I have is a brain and I chose to use it. It's terrifying how few people use their brains to ask important questions such as, why are we still using the same treatment for cancer we were more than 70 years ago? In 1957 we had the pill for birth control, 1962 the launch of the first communications satellite, 1967 we landed on the moon, 1973 the cell phone and magnetic resonance imaging or (MRI), 1978 In-Vitro Fertilization, 1984 DNA Fingerprinting, and finally in 1969 the internet was created and finally commercialised 1995. These are just some of the medical and technological advances spawned from the last 70 years, yet cancer treatment remains the same? If you are as shocked by this as I was you should be, because after billions of dollars and decades of research we have fuck all to show for it!

As for formal qualifications, I have learned that doctors and specialists who would recommend chemotherapy and radiation as a treatment for cancer with cancer-causing agents would put it to better use by wiping their ass. Many friends over the years have graduated with degrees in their chosen field and when it came time to get a job all they were asked was what experience did they have? Currently, many of them are packing boxes in a factory or doing something other than what they studied, demonstrating the real-world value of qualifications and that for most student's university is just a scam to get students into debt early in their lives. What doctors and oncologists won't tell you is that the vast majority would not get chemotherapy or radiation themselves if they were terminally ill, which is exactly what was shown in a study by Stanford University School of Medicine by VJ Periyakoli, MD clinical associate professor of medicine and lead author of the study. The study showed that 88.3% of the doctors surveyed would choose a no-code status, which means do not resuscitate than subject themselves to life-prolonging treatments like chemotherapy if they had a similar terminal illness as their patients, and the majority of doctors that said this were radiologists, radiation oncologists, surgeons and orthopaedists. So ask yourself why would you listen to their advice when they wouldn't do it for themselves? They are happy telling people such as yourself to continue treatment, that's because they do not have the same emotional investment as they do with themselves or their loved ones. It's like the treatment of your disease is like a business transaction, where the number one rule is to leave emotion at the door, there are heaps of professions that adopt this philosophy where less emotion is best for the business but there is also a line you don't cross and we are at the point where doctors have crossed it.

If you are looking for validation in the mainstream media on the issues raised in this book then don't bother, they won't come up and if they do it will be an opportunity for the media to ambush them in an attempt to publically discredit them.

The media always treat people who challenge the norms in our society this way all because they did not accept the narrative being forced down their throats. If you are looking for the government to intervene then forget that too, corporations like Big Pharma have them in their pocket, these people will never be held accountable for their atrocities and they won't see a jail cell either. So the only tool we can use to work out fact from fiction is to start using our heads and start asking the right questions and weigh the answers we get on the balance of probability. We must train our brains to see past the bullshit and glitter that we are fed daily and learn adapt to a new way of living, we must break free from the brainwashing and the daily programming that we all grew up on because billions have been spent learning how to sell us the lie that we all believe.

Corporations are the real players in this world, not governments, governments are only here to police us in case we act out on the crap they sell us. We have created a system where if people outwardly talk about issues such as Genetically Modified Organisms (GMO), fluoridated water, vaccinations, Chemtrails (Geoengineering program) and population control that it seems like insanity even though these are going on right now! David Icke who has been ridiculed for openly speaking about issues like these has said the fear tactics they use are problem, reaction, solution, which is strange because if you relate this to the current cancer issue that is exactly what you see. Corporations create toxic products which we use because we are told they are safe, people then get sick with cancer and other medical conditions and in their desperation for answers, people seek the advice of their doctor.

The doctor tells them to take a drug made by another pharmaceutical company and the patient remains under the illusion that the drug will work. They take the drug which hides the symptoms of the problem and people think they are getting better until they are worse, and the next thing they know they are on their death bed wondering how the fricken hell all of this happened so quickly and the answer is "perception management". These dangers were there the whole time and most people choose not to see them so with the combination of misplaced trust, bad advice and willful ignorance its no wonder this was the outcome.

In an article by The Guardian in Australia a coroner by the name of Audrey Jamieson spoke at the International Medicine in Addiction conference and said that in Victoria 82% of all overdose deaths were due to prescription medications by drugs like opioids for pain management. It also said that anti-depressants and antipsychotics were highly implicated but also Benzodiazepines which are tranquillizer drugs like Valium and Xanax which were lethal if mixed with alcohol, illegal drugs, opioids and antidepressants. According to the ABC in an article posted on their website dated the 19th of December 2017 by Shalailah Medhora titled "Pharmaceutical's officially more of a problem than illicit drugs, report finds" begs the question, exactly what is being done about the misuse of prescription medications by more than 1 million Australians? And now we are being told to trust the COVID 19 vaccine? Its just another drug! Chemotherapy and radiation are just another prescription drug recommended by your oncologist and if over the counter drugs are having this kind of impact then just imagine what cancer drugs must be doing worldwide. Our use and abuse of legal drugs is something that desperately needs our attention and the death toll is climbing alongside big pharma's profits.

This growing problem leaves the death toll of terrorists and third world extremists in the dust, yet when 911 happened and these terrorists killed 2,996 people it was the prelude to an invasion of the Middle East that the American people did not want. In that moment of vulnerability and desperation, the political powers exploited the state of shock people were in to sell them a lie that to this day they are still paying for. So imagine for a second if these terrorists killed 47,600 people what the ramifications would be? Well according to the National Institute of Drug Abuse in 2017 that's exactly how many people died on prescription opioids alone which involved drugs with methadone, heroin and other synthetic narcotics like fentanyl.

If terrorists were responsible for 47,600 deaths the US and all of their allies would have gone into the Middle East and wiped them off the planet. Yet the pharmaceutical industry who has killed more people than most wars in our history continues to do so with impunity. How can this be?

I do not address the issues here lightly and after 10 years of researching what I can only describe as truthology, which is the study of truth, you quickly realize that it can only be done effectively by researching both sides of an argument before formulating a valid opinion, otherwise a person's opinion on something they know nothing about is about as useful as a penis to a nun.

All jokes aside, I can say with no regrets that even if the message here is not received well by the reader I would like to think that there is something to learn for everyone, and if people would only question things more often and not blindly accept what they see and hear at face value then I would be content that my work is done. After 5 years of looking after my father and another 5 researching and putting this book together the work presented here will shock and contradict your doctor's advice when it comes to cancer causation and its treatment. After seeing everything my father went through and everything I learned along the way I asked myself many times, how could I not share it with others? I won't lie when I say that people can make it really hard for you to like them, but even these kinds of people I write this for. Most would agree that killing people is wrong, but I think that letting people die because they were ignorant to what is in this book isn't any better, and why this nagging thought in the back of my head said that I had to do this even if it had the potential to change a single life.

It has taken 3 years to write this book and what I have learned in that time on the subject of cancer boggles the mind, I didn't want to write a book like those rags to riches self-help books where after 200 pages you still can't work out how the hell someone made their first million, then you realize they just did by selling a million copies. What I wanted to give people is something real and practical that was easy to understand but also had my experience with cancer and doctors. When I began looking for cancer treatments other than chemo and radiation, it didn't take long to realize that with a bit of effort you can find dozens if you know where to look, and without harmful side effects.

My father was critical in me realizing a certain truth about cancer and that the biggest obstacle to overcoming it was not in finding a natural or alternative treatment, it was getting my father to ignore his doctor's advice by changing the way he thought about his condition. What people don't realize is that we don't need to hear the official story for anything anymore because it has been dictated to us our whole lives. What we need to do now is open our eyes and our minds to other possibilities and explore the other side of everything we have been led to believe. We must question and challenge our current worldview without fear of ridicule and rejection if we are to find our salvation, that said I bring you Unlocking the Secrets of Cancer which I hope for you is one step closer to that salvation.

PART I

CHAPTER 1: CANCER THE MYSTERY DISEASE

My first taste of the cancer conspiracy was in early 2010 with a documentary called "Cancer: The Forbidden Cures" which was written and directed by Massimo Mazzucco, being a documentary buff and not watching much mainstream TV I was desperate for new material so I thought I'd watch it seeing as I knew nothing on the subject. The documentary was old but the story was all there, and it did well to pique my interest in the subject of cancer causation and how conventional treatment has failed us over the last 100 years.

About 6 months later in late August my mother and father got my sister and me in the loungeroom and told us that my father had Non-Small Cell Lung Cancer (NSCLC), which is where it grows slowly but can become more aggressive and that he needed treatment ASAP. No time is a good time for cancer, but his diagnosis was particularly bad timing because they had just started a huge renovation on the house we were in. When my parents told my sister and me about his condition I initially thought that they were separating. Things had been bad for years with money problems and my father's attitude towards life in general which had been the source of many arguments where my mother's yelling and screaming could suck the life out of anyone standing in the same room. Since I was old enough to push a lawnmower I had always been there to help with the problems my parents were having even at a very young age, this soon became a dependency for me to do things that should not be expected of a child. At some point, this had driven a wedge between my father and me and I felt as if he resented me as my sister could never do anything wrong, and the older I got the less interested he became in our family. Once my grandparents asked him "do you ever tell your kids you love them?".

His answer to this was, no I'm not a homo! Yep, that old chestnut, he actually believed that if you told your son you love him then it makes you less of a man. I guess he was just doing what his father did to him and thought that's how you raise kids. It's safe to say that my father had a bad attitude about most things and according to my mother he was never like this when they were younger. This was a strange thing for me to hear because I could never recall a time when he was any different. I always said that he was a man born tired because he always wanted to do things until it came time to do them. I asked him once what was so bad in his life that made him this way? All he said to me was "Too many hard knocks." After hearing this I thought if this is how he sees his own life how am I going to get him to choose it and beat his cancer when he is acting like an empty shell with nothing to live for?

Even he knew that cancer was a death sentence and if the surgery which is what was being explored at the time went bad then he would be looking at some pretty aggressive treatment. At the time I didn't know that surgery was just as bad as chemo and radiation, so I didn't make a fuss about it, but I had remembered the documentary I watched about 6 months earlier and said to my parents that before he decides anything both of them have to watch it. I knew for a fact that my father wouldn't listen to me, but maybe he would listen to my mother, so I got both to watch the documentary and hoped for a lightbulb moment. My mother's reaction was more significant than my father's considering what I had just shown them, but neither of them thought of it as a serious documentary because it wasn't on mainstream TV, they said to me "if all of this is true then why isn't it all over the news?" The system had brainwashed them well and I quickly realized that my biggest obstacle would be convincing them that conventional treatment would eventually kill him no matter what his oncologist said. Even though I knew little at the time the documentary alone was compelling enough for me not to get chemotherapy and ask a shitload more questions while exploring other options.

I find it interesting that many people who have diseases like cancer cannot tell you much about them considering the impact it is having on their lives, it just goes to show that we have relied on the opinions of doctors far too much when we are afflicted with medical conditions. When it comes to cancer few patients know the things that will make their condition better or worse, so by understanding what the underlying causes may be and the mechanisms that fuel its growth, hopefully, you can start making the right choices sooner rather than later.

Puzzled like most people I set out to find the answers in an attempt to help my father and if I had learned anything from the documentary it was that it would not end at surgery and chemotherapy. Cancer is such a full-on and complex subject that it would be impossible to cover everything here, but I like to think I picked some of the juicer things for you to sink your teeth into as they are truly shocking in their essence.

People's memories are inherently short and to do some of the world's greatest minds justice I decided to rekindle some of the lessons we have forgotten.

As famously put by Graham Hancock "humans are a species with amnesia" and most of us feel deep down that there is something terribly wrong in this world, the reason people feel this way is because they are right and it is not a matter of perspective, we have forgotten some of the most important lessons that some of the world's most influential leaders have tried to teach us. We are currently on a crash course that we seem destined to repeat because collectively we won't wake up and demand the change we need. Instead, we prefer to dumb ourselves down through constant entertainment, medication, and distraction.

So if you are one of these people who thinks that this is all just a bunch of made-up horse shit just to sell a book then I respect your healthy scepticism, but ignoring the message here will have dire consequences sooner or later. So before you judge a book by its cover ask yourself, what do you really know about cancer, and are your opinions informed and valid?

What is Cancer?

By definition, cancer is a systemic metabolic disease that results in uncontrolled cell division leading to malignant growth producing a tumour or mass. When I first looked into cancer I realized early on that most doctors never actually explain what your cancer is or how you may have got it. Ask most people what cancer is and immediately they think of a tumour, which doesn't tell you much other than it's a lump in uncomfortable place. Cancer and other diseases are the result when your body's metabolism is out of equilibrium, there are many reasons for how this could occur but the worst thing you could do is try to put it all down to a single cause or say that it is genetic when there are so many factors that could have contributed to your disease. For example, smoking increases your risk of lung cancer but most people don't know that just as many non-smokers get it as well, therefore smoking is a contributing factor and not the whole picture.

Cancer is a pro-inflammatory condition and there are endless things that can cause inflammation and sabotage your immune system so, therefore, it can be argued that cancer can be caused by anything that attacks thc integrity of your immune system and causes inflammation. There are over 100 diseases that fall into the category of cancer but the most common ones are those that form tumours called carcinomas, they originate from the epithelial cells which are the inner and outer layer of cells that make up all tissues in and outside of the body. Cancers of the blood like leukaemia do not form solid tumours, instead, they originate in the bone marrow that makes blood and crowds out normal blood cells. Leukaemia produces large amounts of abnormal white blood cells which then creates a host of problems like getting oxygen, controlling bleeding and fighting off infection. Cancer can occur anywhere in the body because different cells types make up the body. When cancer is benign its means that the tumours are non-cancerous and can often be removed by surgery posing no real threat. When cancer is malignant it refers to the primary location of cancer and it also means that it can invade other tissues. This process is called metastasis and results in tumours forming in other areas of the body and is by far the most dangerous phase for someone with cancer, these are referred to as secondary cancers. Even though a patient's cancer may have metastasized into other tissues, the cancer is still referred to as primary cancer which caused the metastasis. Metastasis can go anywhere in the body and if ignored or treated poorly the patient will most likely die. When my father had lung cancer it metastasized to his lymph nodes, brain, liver, and pancreas, this is the time to worry because it's when cancer patients are at their most vulnerable as most cancer deaths occur by metastasis, not primary cancer.

Cancer is not homogenous, meaning that there could be several variations within a population of cells that make up a tumour or mass, this makes treatment difficult in a way because there is no telling how each variation will respond to the treatment your doctor gives you. This is also why chemo and radiation have low success rates, the treatments given are broad and not specific to killing different cancer cell types. This results in your oncologist doing mostly guesswork rather than actual science because their approach is just to give you whatever you respond to as cancer is seen as a death sentence anyway. Cancer starts with the nuclei within a cell, the nuclei houses the DNA and therefore the genes within that cell. DNA is the blueprint that tells a cell what it should be, but the cell is so much more complex than just a place to store genetic information. DNA tells the cell how to make a copy of itself and even when the cell should die, this is a process called apoptosis which is an essential phase to all healthy cells in the cell cycle. However, cancer defies the logic of the cell cycle and operates outside of the bodies normal controls, mutations caused by chemicals, radiation or by some other means damages the DNA within a cell making it reproduce in an uncontrolled way. Some of the latest research has found that not all cells can become cancerous, stem cells which are present in all tissue types can become cancer which are known as Cancer Stem Cells (CSC), or the Mother Stem Cell, which we will go into more detail later.

For cancer to be detected by an MRI a cluster of cells needs to be at least 1 billion cells large which depending on the cell type and location may already be quite advanced. What's disturbing is what happens just before you get an MRI to determine how big and where your cancer is. The diagnoses phase demonstrates just how ignorant doctors can be when it comes to cancer and how they treat it. Before you get an MRI patients are told to drink a Glucose solution (sugar) with a radioisotope (radiation) as a type of marker to highlight where and how big the cancer is. This is called a contrast screen and after waiting a short time cancer absorbs the sugar with the radioisotope making it light up like a Christmas tree during the scan, which sounds perfectly normal, right? Well, it's not! First of all, they just put radiation into you which is known to damage DNA and can cause all sorts of cancer, but most importantly if there is one thing that no cancer patient should have its sugar. Sugar is cancer's primary fuel and promotes inflammation in an acidic environment. But what if you are hospitalized due to your condition? Surely you would be on a specialized menu without sugar otherwise your cancer would get worse? Well, your not, you are given the same menu as everyone else, have you ever heard people complaining about how shit hospital food is? Saying things like this crap will kill me! Well if you have cancer and are not on a controlled diet then they are not exaggerating. In fact, before chemotherapy and radiation, you are told the complete opposite by your oncologist and the hospital's dietician. You are told to increase your calorie intake no matter where you get those calories from, so eating shit food is encouraged because their only concern is for you to put on weight because the one thing they do admit treatment kills is your appetite. My father was told to eat pizza, ice cream, pie and chips, drink coke cola you name it, their only concern was to increase his caloric intake and his protein content, so if you're in doubt about this just ask them and see what they say. To read about it here is one thing but seriously I challenge you to ask your oncologist or dietician the logic behind their reasoning and see how they react. This is just one example of how contradicting the advice and treatment for cancer is and once you understand a few basic things about how cancer works and what makes it worse you will start to grasp the scope of how ignorant most doctors are.

So now that we understand some of the basics about what cancer is let's move on to some of the most common types of cancer because one of these may apply to you and will help you better understand your condition and some of the things you could be doing to help your body heal.

The 5 Most Common Types of Cancer

Here we will look into the 5 most common types of cancer which combined just happen to make up 50% of all cancer incidence, we will also look at a few statistics to get an idea of what the cancer incidence and mortality rates are in Australia, but they are no better worldwide.. The statistics I am about to show you on these 5 cancer types are from Cancer Australia which is a government website.

Though the statistics from this source should not be fully trusted we can use the incidence rate of these statistics as a baseline for the annual increase for cancer in Australia.

Skin Cancer

Skin cancer is among the most common type of cancer and occurs when the DNA is damaged in the skin cells by overexposure from UV rays like sunlight, tanning beds and even multiple X-rays which use radiation waves.

Every year come summertime a real sense of fear is instilled into the public from the National Cancer Institute and the Cancer Council Australia about the sun and skin cancer. The truth is that sunlight will not give you skin cancer, 20–30 mins a day has many health benefits like the production of Vitamin D which is essential for boosting your immune system and for general health and wellbeing. Its overexposure that can give you skin cancer, people working on their tan lines to be as beautiful as they can be unprotected for 4 hours straight on a 30-degree day, that can give you skin cancer. There is also a lot of controversy around sunscreens causing cancer due to the chemical filler's used in these products, where oxybenzone seems to be centre stage. Sunscreens also contain avobenzone, octisalate, octocrylene, homosalate and octinoxate all chemicals suspected in causing harm. Though there currently exists no hard scientific studies that conclusively say that sunscreens cause cancer the warning signs are numerous. In a study called "*Dermatological and environmental toxicological impact of the sunscreen ingredient oxybenzone/benzophenone-3*" by Joseph C Di Nardo MS and Craig A Downs at the Haereticus Environmental Laboratory in the USA, they mention that even the Centre for Disease Control in their fourth national report on human exposure to environmental chemicals showed that 97% of their test subjects had traces of oxybenzone in their urine. It further added that scientists have reported oxybenzone in waterways and fish species worldwide and said that oxybenzone when combined with chlorine and other chemicals produce hazardous waste products that are released into the waterways which go into a feedback loop where the fish we eat is contaminated with the chemical and the water treatment protocols we have do not effectively remove the chemical from our tap water. So basically you're eating contaminated fish and drinking sunscreen in your tap water. The environmental impacts of this chemical are just as bad, ranging from a wide variety of toxic reactions in organisms from coral bleaching to mortality.

So here is a simple question, why would chemicals in sunscreen be toxic to the environment but not you and your internal environment? There's no reason its not! Just because science hasn't found the answer yet doesn't make it any less dangerous. The question people need to start asking is who funds these studies that defend the use of a chemical when the scientific community agrees that the exact mechanisms of how it affects human life and other organisms are largely unknown, yet it's deemed to be safe!?

You will soon learn that the scientific community and the regulating authorities generally agree that if a substance has an unknown effect on human health then it is presumed to be safe which is why many of the things you buy at the supermarket may be causing you harm, just like oxybenzone in your sunscreen. Maybe the real reason toxic chemicals like oxybenzone is not getting the attention it deserves is that the products it's in are endorsed by the anti-cancer establishment like the Cancer Council of Australia. Can you imagine the ramifications if it was found that the anti-cancer establishment promoted the use of products that cause cancer? Then again, I have seen representatives of the Cancer Council sell confectionary at hospital's to promote their cause, which if you knew how cancer reacts to sugar as you do now, then it would be no different to me running a gym for weight loss and selling chocolate pudding to my customers on the way out, what a way to guarantee business.

If you go to the Cancer Councils website in the top left corner of the home page is their sun-smart warning which literally says "Sun Protection Required", which is an interesting choice of words, are they informing us or telling us? It would be like me saying reading this book is required, it doesn't make you feel like your choice is important, does it?

Skin cancer is the third most common type of cancer in Australia and according to Cancer Australia in 2020 it was estimated that there were 16,221 new cases of melanoma and an estimated 1,375 resulting deaths. As a precaution against overexposure try wearing more clothes at the beach, in the old days it was considered unseemly to walk at the beach half-naked and so the skin cancer incidence rate was significantly lower. Because things have moved on since the Middle Ages I realise that is not always practical to be fully clothed on a 30-degree day at your favourite beach. With golden sand and crystal clear water, it's better enjoyed in your favourite swimsuit even if what they are wearing looks more like an eye patch.

Fortunately, alternatives do exist, organic cold-pressed coconut oil can be used as a mild sunscreen if you're looking to go organic and it can also hydrate your skin. Alternatively don't just buy the cheapest sunscreen at the supermarket, many are loaded with toxic rubbish and not just oxybenzone but avobenzone, octisalate, octocrylene, homosalate and octinoxate all of which are endocrine disruptors that disrupt or mimic hormones, oxybenzone has also been linked to Hirschsprung's disease which is a problem with your large intestine.

What you are ideally looking for in a good sunscreen is a mineral sunscreen without a chemical filler, mineral sunscreens deflect light away from the skin which has proven to be just as effective if not better than the chemical ones. Look for a mineral sunscreen in either a cream or lotion and not a spray, the best part about these sunscreens is that the cost is virtually the same, so you are getting a far safer and healthier product for the same cost. If you struggle to find any of these try online or at your local health food store.

Caution: Non-mineral based sunscreens basically form a skin over your skin which makes sweating difficult, this means that toxins that would have been normally excreted through your skin during sweating stay in the body longer increasing your toxic load and putting more biological stress on the body, avoid these types of sunscreens.

Early Detection

Statistically speaking although melanoma is the most common type of cancer it is not the most fatal, symptoms may include a change in the texture of skin at the site and there is usually no pain.

Early signs include skin, freckles and moles changing in size, shape and colour over several weeks and months; the site will usually feel different to the touch.

Prostate Cancer

The prostate is a gland that makes the fluid that forms part of the semen which surrounds the urethra, the tube where semen and urine come out. Urine flows out of the bladder and leaves your body through your urethra so if your prostate is enlarged you may have trouble peeing and may need a urinary catheter.

This instinctually makes every man weep because the male pee hole is small for a reason and big things like catheters are not supposed to be shoved up there. It is suggested that males get a prostate examination between the ages of 40-50 depending on your level of risk. According to Cancer Australia in 2020 it was estimated that there were 16,741 new cases of prostate cancer where 3,152 were estimated to have died.

Some of the things you could be doing now in response to your prostate cancer is concentrating on unhealthy habits such as smoking and consuming alcohol, also if you have high levels of calcium or are obese then these risk factors and are likely to contribute to your condition. Diet is extremely important, but we will get into the details later of what you should be eating to help with your condition.

People with prostate cancer are sometimes told that the cause for prostate cancer is genetic, the genes they are referring to are:

- RNASEL, formerly known as HPCI

- BRCA1 and BRCA2, which have also been linked to breast and ovarian cancer in women
- MSH2, MLH1, and other DNA mismatch repair genes HOXB13

However, this may not be the case at all as I will explain in chapters to come.

Mainstream science also says that age is another risk factor which makes sense for all cancer types and not just prostate cancer, which we will also explore later.

Early Detection

Surprisingly many men die with prostate cancer but not from it, it's one of the few cancer types that can stay under the radar unless it has progressed to an aggressive state. Some of the early signs of prostate cancer are burning or pain during urination, difficulty urinating, or trouble starting and stopping while urinating, more frequent urges to urinate at night, loss of bladder control, decreased flow or velocity of urine stream, blood in the urine (hematuria), blood in semen, difficulty getting an erection (erectile dysfunction), painful ejaculation, swelling in legs or pelvic area, numbness or pain in the hips, legs or feet, bone pain that doesn't go away which may lead to fractures. Many of these symptoms can also be bladder related and may not be prostate cancer so be thorough with your doctor and their diagnosis.

Breast Cancer

Breast cancer primarily occurs in women but in rare cases men as well, the breast is made up of lobules and ducts, lobules make breast milk and the ducts carry the milk to the nipple. Close to the breasts are lymph nodes which make up the lymphatic system, their function is to trap harmful bacteria, free radicals and cancer cells where they neutralise them with enzymes before they can harm tissues and vital organs. Swollen lymph nodes in the breast indicate that they are working and not necessarily cancerous, a lymph node may be swollen due to the many toxins it has trapped and trying to neutralise. What's alarming about this is that many women instructed by their doctors have been told to go get a mammogram for early breast cancer detection because these areas of the breast appear firm to the touch due to the inflammation.

The mammogram then puts 4.4 psi which would feel like 50 pounds of weight on their breasts putting pressure on the lymph node and then bursting it releasing all the harmful toxins it was trying to neutralize back into the bloodstream which can cause cancer in the breast. It's fair to say that in many cases where a mammogram is used women have had their condition worsened by the diagnostic procedure due to this lack of understanding by their doctor, fortunately here in Australia safer methods of diagnosis are currently being used.

There are 2 common types of breast cancer, non-invasive and invasive, both originate in the lobules or ducts, non-invasive stays where it originated and the other spreads to the remaining breast tissues.

According to Cancer Australia in 2020 it was estimated that there were 19,974 which has resulted in approximately 3,031 deaths. Common causes of breast cancer may be from things like deodorants and cosmetics where their ingredients are adding to the bio-accumulation of toxic chemicals and heavy metals over time resulting in cancer and other chronic diseases. According to Professor Philippa D Darbre at Reading University our bodies, specifically the breasts, are polluted with a cocktail of all sorts of toxic chemicals leading to endocrine disruption and has the absolute potential for breast cancer to develop.

The biggest risk factors that are said to contribute to breast cancer are:

- The BRCA1 and BRCA2 (BRCA1/2) genes
- Diet/Alcohol/Radiation
- Obesity
- Hormonal effects – Lifetime exposure to estrogen, contraception vs hormone replacement therapy, giving birth and breastfeeding
- Environmental Chemicals – Herbicides and pesticides, non-stick pans, plastics and detergents
- Personal care products – Aluminium from deodorants, antiaging products, UV filters and parabens are just some

A big argument in the mainstream scientific community about cancer being genetic relies largely on the loss of function in the BRCA1 and BRCA2 genes being the cause of breast and even prostate cancer, even though they cannot tell you what the catalyst for this loss of function is. It could have been any of the things just mentioned but because the exact mechanism of its pathology is largely unknown they just say it's genetic.

Early Detection

Early signs of breast cancer may include swelling of all or part of the breast even if no distinct lump is felt, skin irritation or dimpling, breast or nipple pain, nipple retraction, redness, scaliness, or thickening of the nipple or breast skin, nipple discharge (other than breast milk).

Lung Cancer

The lung is structured like an upside-down tree where the thickest part is called the bronchi which is connected to your trachea or throat. The bronchi branch's off into the lungs until the finest point where air sacs are attached; these are called alveoli, which have the task of exchanging gases such as oxygen when you breathe in and carbon dioxide when you breathe out. Lung cancer occurs when the bronchi or alveoli are obstructed by the cancerous growth interfering with the exchange of gases causing breathing difficulties wherein advanced stages can lead to hospitalisation. The cancer forms in the epithelial cells, the inner and outer layer of cells in the lung tissue blocking the passage for oxygen to get into the body.

There are two main types of lung cancer, non-small cell (NSCLC) and small cell (SCLC), 85-90% of lung cancer is non-small cell lung cancer, and this is when cancer starts slow and originates in the outer part of the lung before it has time spread. Small cell lung cancer occurs in the bronchi and is usually fast-growing and more aggressive. According to cancer research UK in 2012 an alarming 1.59 million people died from lung cancer worldwide and occurred in more deprived areas. In 2014, 35,900 people died in the UK of lung cancer which equates to 98 deaths every single day. In 2020 Cancer Australia estimates that there were approximately 13,258 new lung cancer cases which resulted in 8,641 deaths. The mainstream scientific and medical community believe that there are some genetic components to lung cancer but they are not inherited ones passed down from generation to generation.

Early Detection

Some of the early symptoms of lung cancer may include chest discomfort or pain, a cough that doesn't go away or gets worse over time, trouble breathing, wheezing,
blood in sputum (mucus coughed up from the lungs), hoarseness, trouble swallowing, loss of appetite, weight loss for no known reason, feeling very tired, swelling in the face and/or veins in the neck.

Bowel Cancer

Bowel cancer is also known as colorectal cancer and occurs mostly in the lining of the large bowel. Small growths called polyps which are tissues that have blood vessels in them are found in the colon, nose or uterus become cancerous and eventually malignant.

The conventional solution to this is endoscopic treatment, which is a specialised rod in the rectum to surgically remove the polyps.

According to cancer research UK in 2012 694,000 people worldwide were estimated to have died from bowel cancer and like lung cancer those who lived in deprived regions of the world were most at risk.

According to Cancer Australia in 2020 it was estimated that there were 15,494 new bowel cancer cases which resulted in approximately 5,322 deaths.

The 3 most common inherited syndromes associated with bowel cancer are:

- Hereditary Non-Polyposis Colorectal Cancer (HNPCC) also known as Lynch Syndrome
- Familial adenomatous polyposis (FAP) and
- MYH-Associated Polyposis (MAP)

Because the mainstream solution is to surgically remove these polyps there is some cause for concern even though surgery is the safest out of all 3 conventional treatments for cancer. What your oncologist doesn't tell you is that surgery has many hidden risks that may worsen your condition but we will explore these later.

Early Detection

There are different types of colon polyps where only a handful can cause symptoms or signs of being potential cancer, such as red blood or black stool sample which would have most people worried. There is also paleness, fatigue, pain in the abdomen, abdominal discomfort, excessive gas, anaemia and unexplained weight loss.

The trouble with the diagnosis of this type of cancer is that due to the nonspecific symptoms it could be a whole range of chronic medical conditions like stress, ulcers in the stomach, Irritable Bowel Syndrome (IBS), parasitic infection, candida infection, haemorrhoids and a bunch of others. The only reliable diagnostic test to determine the cause is gastroscopy or colonoscopy.

If you have 1 of these 5 common types of cancer then hopefully by now you know a little more about them than you did before, however, there is something sinister in these statistics about the expected survival rate of up to 5 years. There's a reason why these statistics only go for 5 years and no longer and that's because approximately 2.1% of people survive beyond that 5-year threshold after conventional treatment. Cancer Australia is a government website and they are dead wrong about the survivability of cancer once a person undergoes conventional treatment. The reason this information on survivability is misleading is because of how a cancer survivor is defined, for example: If you were diagnosed with cancer on the 1st of January 2010 and you died on the 2nd of January 2015, statistically you are a cancer survivor even though you are dead. This is exactly why government statistics cannot be fully trusted; they are manipulated and used to sell the lie that conventional treatment works because cancer treatments alone make more than 200 billion dollars every year, some of which is donated to certain political parties to pass laws favourable to the companies selling the treatment.

People don't realize that scientists working in government or for the pharmaceutical industry can manipulate their studies to produce the results they want. This is done to sell the masses the narrative that conventional treatment works and that no other option exists.

Even if mainstream science had a study that showed conventional treatment treating a patients cancer with no harmful side effects and could extend their life beyond 5 years it couldn't be trusted based solely on the fact that the study's results could have been manipulated to show exactly that.

The real question becomes how can we trust authority on anything? If you ask most people, do you trust the government? Most sane people would say no! Yet why do these same people believe the data the government supports if they don't trust them? This is a perplexing dilemma and huge contradiction in behavour. There is so much information out there today who can you trust? The information we get on a day to day basis is so volatile that one minute something is good for us and the next it's completely different.

Another example is how statistics are manipulated to convince the public on the cancer incidence rates between the years 1982 to 2017. In Australia, cancer incidence has progressively increased from 47,440 cases each year to 134,174, but because of national standardisation they are expressed in every 100,000 as opposed to every 10,000, this is done so visually the graph doesn't seem as significant as it really is.

However, if we expressed the same data by changing the national standard to 500,000, which is roughly one in every 50 people, the same data would appear as a straight horizontal line across the graph which visually would look like nothing at all, even though cancer incidence has nearly tripled in just 35 years.

If cancer incidence has grown so rapidly in Australia and you have experts telling everyone it's genetic how the hell do they get away with this when they cannot even tell you the reason for this genetic malfunction? To say it's genetic without sufficient explanation is like giving an answer that's not an answer, and the ones that do that best are politicians. Even the Cancer Councils website says that Australia has 17,500 more people die each year than only 30 years ago. Compared to COVID deaths in Australia this is infinitely more significant and yet you hear nothing about it! Furthermore, if the data on mortality took into consideration a 10-year timeframe instead of a 5-year timeframe, then perhaps the figures would show the 2.1% survivability rate which would put cancer mortality closer to the rate of incidence and the true effectiveness of conventional treatment would be exposed.

According to Cancer Research UK, it was estimated that in 2012 there were 14.1 million new cases of cancer worldwide and in the same year there were 8.2 million cancer-related deaths, that's more than 16 times the death toll of the Iraq Wars which occurred over 7 years! Logic 101 says that we are clearly doing something wrong in the world to have modern disease increase this much and these are only the cancer figures, can you imagine all of the other diseases?

The genetic argument for cancer causation is a poor one and does not adequately explain a death toll of this magnitude, it is just a theory like evolution, and a fallacy that allows the continuation of a dangerous practice all because it's profitable. So let's put their theory to the test and take a brief look at our history to see if we can find a genetic cause for modern cancer causation that reflects what we see today.

CHAPTER 2: CANCER & GENETICS! IT'S JUST A THEORY!

Have you ever heard of the human genome project? Mainstream science had led us to believe that with the complete mapping of human DNA that the war on cancer would be won. The aim of the project was to sequence all 3 billion base pair combinations including the 20-25,000 human genes that science believes causes diseases like cancer. The project started in 1990 and finished in April 2003, 2003! It's 2021, a whopping 18 years later and what do we have to show for it? Fuck all! The project did find the BRCA1 gene in 1994 and the BRCA2 gene in 1995 which are said to be hereditary genes for breast and prostate cancer, so what revolutionary treatments have resulted from these discoveries? Nothing, in fact, scientists are not even sure how these genes work, so all we have is the mainstream scientific community stringing us along to find another carrot they can dangle in front of us. Do you think it's a coincidence that every time you hear about some cancer breakthrough on the news or the radio that human trials won't start until a few years from the announcement, and then a decade later were back to square one? It's not a coincidence...

We are still approaching and treating cancer the way we did 100 years ago and that approach is based on a profitable system, so why would they change it? Perhaps the answer is simpler than scientists would like to admit and the reason they cannot find a genetic cause for cancer is that there isn't one. More than 100 years have been spent looking for flaws in the cell's DNA and after finding 291 genes which is a little more than 1% of the complete human genome the only prominent gene that science has managed to find is the tumour suppressor gene called P53.

P53 is a tumour protein and is responsible for regulating the cell cycle and it essentially it functions to suppress cancer in multicellular organisms such as humans. Genes are like light switches and they can be turned on or off by things like chemicals, drugs, poor nutrition and other harmful substances, so genetics is not so much the cause of cancer but more like the symptom. Therefore, the catalyst for DNA damage and malfunction could just as easily be an accumulation of harmful substances and not a loss of function due to a person's genes. If you walk over to a light switch and turn it on you don't say that the light came on by itself, the reason it lit up is that you walked over to the switch and turned it on. Therefore, you are the catalyst and without this action, the light would have never come on, well genes and cancer could work the same way.

If you think about this logically, you are expected to believe that science has invested more than 100 years of research into cancer causation with genetics at its core and billions of dollars invested and donated, not to mention the advancements in technology and the only prominent gene to date is the P53 gene? What should shock you is that all of these so-called intelligent scientists perpetuating this genetics rubbish, at no point whatsoever consider that maybe, just maybe there isn't a genetic cause! At least not one that explains cancer incidence rates increasing the way we are seeing it today. Now I'm not saying that some cancers cannot be caused by genetics, because the truth is we don't know. What I am saying is that in the last 10 years of research genetics does not explain why 1 in 2 people get cancer today, it has to be environmental.

This exponential growth means that by the year 2050 cancer incidence rates could easily double, meaning that mainstream science wants us to believe that as we continue to pollute our planet and the things we take from it, that the increase in cancer and other diseases are caused by genetics. Scientists are supposed to have the answers but when it comes to cancer causation it's mostly guesswork and a whole bunch of theories, and theories do not always translate into facts.

The Molecular Theory of Cancer

This is also known as the Somatic Cell Theory of cancer, it consists of 95% of all cancers and has been the prevailing theory of cancer causation for the last 100 years. This theory has largely stayed the same despite modern advancements in technology, which suggests that a limited number of genes causes cancer. There are 3 premises for this theory.

- Cancer occurs within a single cell due to multiple DNA mutations over time degrading the integrity of the cell's DNA.
- The absence of regulatory stimuli which is the default state of cells in multicellular organisms is essentially inactive or in dormancy.
- Cancer is a disease of cell proliferation or the cell cycle.

This theory doesn't sound so bad until you consider the treatment of cancer, which is chemotherapy and/or radiation.

Both of these treatments are known to directly damage DNA and kill all cell types. If this theory says DNA damage causes cancer then why is the treatment of cancer to give you something that they know damages DNA? How can you possibly get better by making you worse?

Conventional treatment under this theory can only result in a feedback loop of cell toxicity where the patient will inevitably die due to the toxic components of the treatment and the body's limited mechanisms for removal.

The Immune System Theory

This is an interesting theory and very compelling in its own right. It states that cancer is an out of control immune response to injury in the body. Just like your immune system responds to a cut and tries to heal it your immune system responds to the internal injury of tissues and cancer is the result. This theory is suggesting that cancer maybe your body's alarm system telling you to stop doing what you are doing because it is causing biological stress and injury. Again, even if the mainstream scientific community subscribed to this theory the conventional treatment of cancer with chemo and radiation annihilates the immune system, and once again contradicts the theories own logic for how cancer is caused and how to effectively treat it.

The Chromosomal Theory of Cancer

This theory is like the somatic cell theory in that it goes back to genetics, where cancer is the result of Aneuploidy. Aneuploidy means there is an error in cell division that results in your cells having the wrong number of chromosomes in their daughter cells. In some cases, there is a missing chromosome, while in others an extra.

Unlike the somatic cell theory that says all cancers should be more or less the same, the chromosomal theory according to genetics researcher Peter Duesberg, professor of molecular and cell biology at the University of California said the following in Scientific America in May 2007.

Even if cancers are from the same tissue, and are generated with the same carcinogen, they are never the same. There is always a cytogenetic and biochemical individuality in every cancer.

This statement renders all current theories on cancer utterly useless! If everyone's cancer is unique to the individual then adopting this one size fits all approach which hasn't worked in the last 100 years is nothing more than guesswork and bad science by the medical profession. Doctors from all specializations should at least be offering patients the option of personalised therapies tailored to each individual. Again, we are back at square one because conventional treatment wouldn't work with this theory without contradicting its fundamental principles.

The Cancer Stem Cell Theory

This is the theory we will be focussing on which is somewhat controversial and it has a lot to say about cancer causation and how cancer is treated. It was once believed that any cell could be a cancer cell, but the theory now is that cancer cells may have a hierarchy like other cells in the body. The evidence for this is quite compelling and has been growing since their discovery in 1994. Science has learned that stem cells that become cancerous do so between their embryonic stage and adult stage, the reason stem cells can become cancerous is that is they are effectively a clean slate and have not been given genetic instruction on what to be yet.

The cancer stem cell (CSC) or mother stem cell is a subpopulation of cells that accounts for roughly 2-3% of a tumours mass and scientists have also learned that when metastasis occurs its due to the cancer stem cell, not the daughter cells. When a chemical or radiation interferes with the DNA of a stem cell it becomes damaged or deranged which produces many daughter cells like it, but not exact, and eventually creates the bulk of a tumour or mass. If you have been unfortunate enough to undergo conventional treatment then you may have heard your oncologist say how well you have responded to treatment from chemo or radiation. In reality, all they have done is kill a bunch of daughter cells which made up the bulk of a tumours mass. Remember, a tumour has to be at least 1 billion cells before a scan can pick it up, so a reduction in tumour mass even to the point where you cannot see it on a scan doesn't mean they have killed it, which is why reoccurrences are so common.

When it came to my father's lung cancer this was the textbook approach on how oncologists treated his cancer, so I know this may be hard to hear but believe me it needs to be heard. This understanding of CSC should have revolutionised the way we treat cancer and how the treatment is administered, but it has had no impact at all, in fact, according to Dr Max Wicha an oncologist and professor of over 30 years at the University of Michigan, he said...

"When a drug like chemotherapy reduces the mass of a tumour by 50% the FDA will approve the drug for active use because it's had an effect even if it doesn't heal the patient"

Scientists have also found that CSC's are also "Chemoresistant", meaning that treatment doesn't kill the CSC, just the daughter cells which goes back to my point on why reoccurrence is so common in conventional treatment.

In a study called "*Cancer Stem Cells (CSCs) in Drug Resistance and their Therapeutic Implications in Cancer Treatment"* by the Soonchunhyang Institute of Medi-bio Science (SIMS) at Soonchunhyang University, Asan in the Republic of Korea, they concluded the following on how CSC's and the effects of conventional therapies:

> *CSCs possess stem cell-like features found in cancer and have important implications for the chemoresistance and cancer relapse, a notion that remains somewhat controversial. With a small subpopulation in the malignant cell pool, the contribution of CSCs is remarkable in cancer therapy, as shown by intensive studies in recent decades. They are resistant to chemotherapy and radiation therapy compared to bulk tumour cells and hence play a crucial role in tumour recurrence after anticancer therapy. To survive following cancer treatment, CSCs seem to be able to manifest several responses such as Epithelial-Mesenchymal Transition (EMT), induction of signalling pathways that regulate self-renewal or influence tumour environments, expression of drug transporters or detoxification proteins, and so forth to protect them from devastating effects caused by therapeutic agents.*

In laymen's terms, conventional treatment is shit, doesn't work and makes it worse!

Put simply CSC's are tough to kill and conventional therapies only make it more resilient and this may have something to do with the fact that it's "Immortal", which means that it does not go through the normal cell cycle and reach "Apoptosis" which is programmed cell death. Every cell in your body has a lifespan and depending on the type of cell it could live for days or years. For example, a stomach lining cell can live for roughly 2 days whereas a bone cell can live as long as 25 to 30 years, so they vary greatly depending on what they are. Cancer cells do not go through this process and can self-renew, the only way CSC can be dealt with is if the DNA that's damaged within the cell is fixed or it is killed by the restoration of the immune system.

Fortunately, there are many organic compounds found in many fruits and vegetables that can target and induce cellular stress to the CSC. A study published in the American Journal of Cancer Research called *"The use of natural products to target cancer stem cells"* by Wesley F Taylor and Ehsan Jabbarzadeh at the Department of Chemical Engineering, at the University of South Carolina in Columbia USA, mentions that there are many natural compounds that could be used in personal therapies and can be used as a "chemopreventive" that do not carry the adverse side effects of conventional chemotherapy.

The 2 most notable polyphenols that were shown to have cytotoxic effects on the CSC in the study were Resveratrol which is found in the skins of grapes and berries and also Curcumin which is a compound found in turmeric, others mentioned were piperine found in black pepper, Dihydrocapsaicin found in many species of red and green pepper which is what gives it its hotness, Vitamin A (retinol) and even Brefeldin A which is found in fungi like Penicillium brefeldianum which was even shown to have anti-cancer potential in leukaemia, colon and prostate cancer.

So in the end what theory is right? Well let's think about it, all have their pros and cons, but science doesn't work like that, science wants to put cancer causation into neat little boxes and find a common underlying cause which theoretically sounds great but practically impossible. So what theory do you like the best? I am more partial to the CSC theory, but even this cannot explain all cancer. I have my own opinion on cancer causation which is very unscientific, obviously because I am not a scientist, but in many respects, you don't need to be to find studies like these, read and interpret them. Personally, based on my experience and given what we currently know about cancer this is my logical observational hypothesis and goes something like this…

It is our current understanding that there are more than 100 different types of cancer and so there might as well be at least 100 corresponding causes none of which are definitively known. So what if the cause of all cancer and modern disease is that the world has put itself into one gigantic toxic feedback loop where toxic substances are entering the body at a rate faster than the body can remove. There are several key arguments that I like to support this hypothesis which I call "The Global Biome Feedback Loop".

All theories on cancer causation agree that cellular stress and DNA damage causes cancerous growth which is exactly what happens if you are exposed to the hundreds of toxic chemicals and heavy metals found in our food, water, air and the rest of our environment today.

The world is made up of many ecosystems that are interconnected even at the local level, an example of this is the deforestation of the Amazon which is also known as the lungs of the planet, it gets that name because of how much oxygen it contributes to the planet, not South America where it is located. The reason older people are more at risk is that when they age the DNA in their cells degrade and loses its integrity, also, the older someone is the greater the bioaccumulation of toxic substances, this convergence results in chronic diseases like cancer. Environmental pollution is on the rise and the protocols for the removal of these harmful pollutants are insufficient, humans eat many species of plants and animals found in these contaminated environments which continue to be polluted. For example, there is so much plastic in the ocean right now that we have literally changed the composition of the ocean from water to water and plastic.

Regulating authorities allow the continued use of products even if there is little to no long term safety studies showing their impact on human health. These products affect us in 2 ways, directly when they are used, and indirectly when they are disposed of, contributing to the pollution of the environment and the species that live within them. There is no known safe level of many chemicals and heavy metals that are in the products sold to everyday consumers, Aluminium is a perfect example. To say that we only get exposed to a small amount of anything when the safe level of exposure is unknown is simply Ludacris!

There is no human on the planet including newborn children that are chemical and heavy metal-free which is why so many people suffer from chronic illnesses, including young children which are more at risk during their developing years.

As our ignorance grows so does our problems and the opportunity to change things before we put ourselves into a situation that we cannot return from grow greater by the day. Cancers ability to self-renew and become immortal is interesting in the sense that technically it can outlive the host which it relies on to grow. Cancer also doesn't spread right away which means that it's giving the person a chance to reverse the damage before it can do more harm, this is actually what Andreas Mortiz said in his book which is titled "Cancer is not a disease - it's a healing mechanism". Although the mainstream medical and scientific community have labelled Andreas Moritz for his so-called pseudo-medical practices, I have personally had good results trying his liver and gallbladder flush which we will get into later.

If we go back to Professor Peter Duesberg on the chromosomal theory of cancer, he practically confirms it. Even if cancers are from the same tissue and are generated with the same carcinogen, they are never the same, there is always a cytogenetic and biochemical individuality in every cancer. Conventional wisdom says this cannot be, but it is often those who challenge the current paradigm that makes the greatest change.

Do you think that we got this far as a species by agreeing all the time? If you think about the dramatic lifestyle and environmental changes we have made in the last 200 years is it a surprise that diseases like cancer are the result? One of the greatest dogmas of our time is that scientists believe that mechanistic medicine is the only kind that works, which is why governments never fund or support complementary or alternative treatments. This was a quote from Rupert Sheldrake author of "The Science Delusion" which is based on the 10 dogmas of science that the mainstream scientific community believe and do not know to be a fact. So ask yourself, why are their beliefs on this subject more important than anyone else's when they have no facts to back them?

Medical science is addressing diseases like cancer in the wrong way, it's so focussed on finding a genetic cause that it's blind, or worse, willful ignorant to any other possibility. If mutations or double-strand breaks in DNA cause cancer then what causes mutations and double-strand DNA breaks? It's well established that many chemicals and heavy metals which are found in common household products that we use on a day to day basis are potentially carcinogenic and cause this exact kind of cellular damage to DNA.

So from here, I would like to take you from fiction to fact, because some of the "facts" in the subjects we are about to cover have been so completely distorted that even experts don't know the difference.

CHAPTER 3: CANCER A MODERN DISEASE

Cancer first got its name from the Greek physician Hippocrates (460-370 BC), who is considered to be the father of all medicine. Hippocrates used the word Carcinos and Carcinoma to describe ulcer forming and non-ulcer forming tumours. Carcinos is the Greek word for crab, the crab reminded Hippocrates of what cancer looks like, the shell representing a mass or tumour where the legs represent it spreading out as cancer often does. Later the Roman physician Celsus in 28-50 BC translated the word Carcinos into cancer which is the Latin word for Crab and the word cancer was born.

Historical data into ancient history shows that people knew about cancer as far back as 2500 years ago. Ask yourself, if cancer is a genetic disease which is a major argument in the medical and scientific community, then why isn't it commonly found in ancient remains? To date, there has only been approximately 200 skeletons and mummies that have shown to have cancer of some kind indicating that it was extremely rare in ancient times. Although cancer was present it was also rarely seen, cultures like the ancient Egyptians, Greeks and Mayans who knew of its existence did not have a cancer incidence rate like we do today. The Greeks in ancient times were among the first to distinguish the difference between benign and malignant cancers and it's difficult to say if there was an actual increase in cancer incidence around this time or the Greeks just got better at diagnosing the condition as their medical understanding advanced.

Ancient man wasn't clueless and for their time they go far beyond the intellectual capacity of an advanced ape scratching their ass trying to keep warm in some dark and dreary cave. Their understanding of nature, the elements, energy and the cosmos in many respects exceeds our knowledge today and could teach a few of these experts just how little they know. A good example of this is the great pyramid of Giza which has 9 sides, not 5 including the base, this can only be seen twice a year during the spring and autumn equinox which is where day and night are of equal length. The pyramid is also 0.05 degrees from true north, which given its scale is an incredible feat, and the latitude that it sits on is 29.9792458 which is the exact number for the speed of light in meters per second (299,792,458 m/s).

Given this information do you really think that whoever built the pyramids of Giza didn't know what they were doing? Or that they were oblivious to architecture, the cosmos, agriculture, medicine and all of the other professions we hold dear today? Of course not! Today you can't even get a guy to tile your bathroom properly, much less build a fucking pyramid of the scale and precision of the Giza pyramid. Only we are stupid enough to measure a person's intelligence and capability by a piece of paper and yet today we think of ourselves as being so much superior to ancient man when we would struggle to replicate many of their feats.

Ancient man's medical understanding was equally impressive and though many natural medicines were practiced for various conditions eliminating the need for complicated surgeries, they even performed a primitive type of brain surgery called trepanation.

Trepanation is considered to be the oldest surgery of its kind and goes back to France around 6500BC. (See Below)

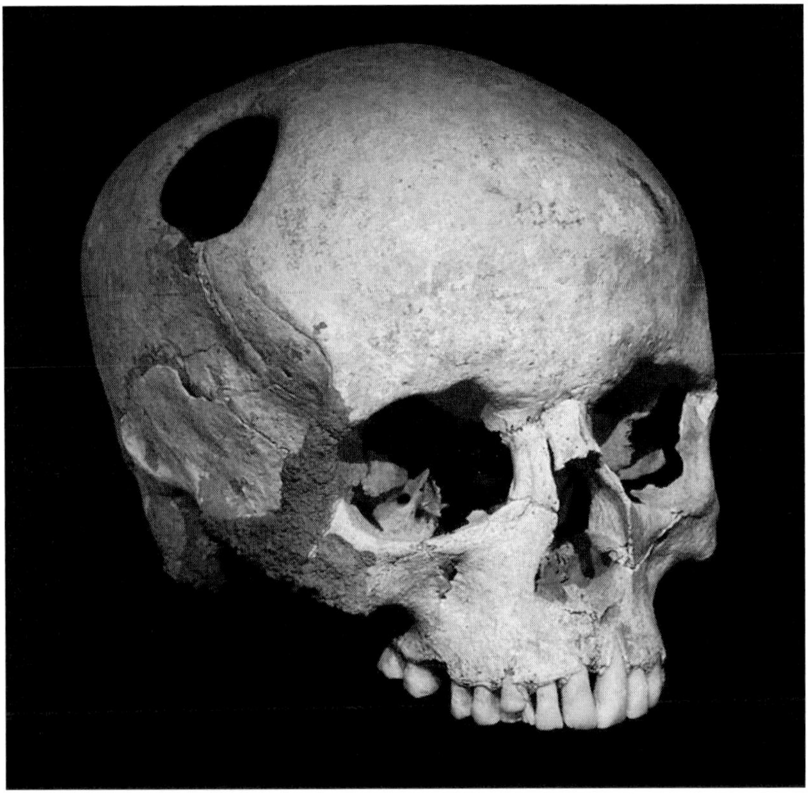

It has also been shown that people subjected to this type of surgery had survived and went on to live for many years after. This says a lot about a so-called primitive culture when modern-day surgeons are practically doing the same thing.

Many diseases were present in the ancient past which had established themselves within wild animal populations, but it wasn't until 11,000 years ago when man developed agriculture that these diseases started to affect human populations. Although the exact origin of many infectious diseases is still unknown today it is thought that diphtheria, influenza A, measles, mumps, pertussis, rotavirus, smallpox and tuberculosis made the transition to humans from domestic animals.

It is also thought that hepatitis B came from Apes and rodents which gave us the plague and typhus, yet funny enough scientists have no idea on the origin of rubella, syphilis, tetanus and typhoid.

In recent times we have learned that the root cause for many diseases is contaminated water supplies and unsanitary living environments. Strangely enough, as we have improved our living standards and sanitised these environments we have reduced the occurrence of infectious diseases, but have seen a rapid increase of chronic diseases like cancer. One of the earliest accounts of cancer was found in the Edwin Smith Papyrus which is dated 1600BC but is said to be referencing another document dated around 3000BC of a tumour in a woman's breast. Studies on thousands of skeletons of Neanderthal man in Europe have yielded few results into the fossil record on cancer incidence and the only thing found to date is the Stetten II skull bone from Stetten, Germany, (35,000 years BP) which provides the only example of a lesion that might be related to a neoplasm (cancer). Another early example of a tumour was found in the femur of a Homo erectus bone, discovered in Java Indonesia, but it was later thought that it might be a benign boney proliferation, which may have been misdiagnosed as myositis ossificans, which is bone tissue that is generated in muscle tissue as a result of trauma or haemorrhage.

Professor Michael R. Zimmerman a paleopathologist which is the study of ancient animal and human remains, with his colleague Rosalie David at the University of Pennsylvania have been studying ancient remains for diseases like cancer particularly in Egypt. The Egyptians are known for their mummification process and have preserved many diseases that would normally be lost due to decomposition. Although other factors are playing into the preservation of ancient diseases, in researching this book Professor Zimmerman was kind enough to point me in the right direction and sent me a document which said the following about other researchers looking for cancer in ancient times.

The group at the Medical College of Virginia in Richmond has examined hundreds of Peruvian and Chilean mummies and has identified only one malignancy, a skeletal muscle tumour (rhabdomyosarcoma) of the face in a young child. This tumour is vanishingly rare in modern populations and may be due to a viral infection.

Professor Zimmerman has also studied more than 100 mummies from upper Egypt using the Walker-Ruffer Rehydration Solution technique, which is where pieces of mummified tissue are rehydrated or softened for postmortem fingerprinting or microscopic examination. His research found that many diseases were present in the remains of the mummies, but only 4 neoplasms (cancer) in total have been found. He went on to say the following.

The virtual absence of malignancies in mummies must be interpreted as indicating their rarity in antiquity, indicating that cancer-causing factors are limited to societies affected by modern industrialisation.

Although we differ in opinion in some things, overall we agree that cancer is a result of modern industrialisation and toxic substances made legal by corporations such as tobacco. Agriculture has changed humans from hunter-gather societies to enormous nations and there has been a tremendous impact in our health along the way, one with consequences that we are just starting to see.

Professor Zimmerman has received a lot of criticism on his findings, even though his research yielded just how uncommon cancer was in the ancient past. These critics are not taking into account that only 50 years ago the cancer incidence rate was 1 in 20 and is now 1 in 2, which is a huge spike and within a person's lifetime. Mainstream arguments for cancer incidence in ancient times usually relies on life expectancy and that people did not live as long as they do today. Cancer affects most people when they are upwards of 50, whereas in ancient times you would have been very lucky to live to the age of 50. However, this doesn’t make sense either, because even if you were 50 years old it would not be equivalent to a 50-year-old today. A 50-year-old today would have accumulated more chemicals and heavy metals in their body than those in the ancient past due to our self-inflicted global pollution problem.

Another argument to make is that cancer found in the ancient past was rare but cancer in children was even rarer! This is validated by more than 12,400 children and adolescents under the age of 20 that were diagnosed with cancer in the US during the year 2000. These child and adolescent cancers seem to occur in three main types which are leukaemia, CNS and brain tumours, and lymphomas.

So ask yourself, why doesn't the same types of cancer or the percentage of cancers appear in the ancient remains of children? I mean if its genetic like the experts claim it should be there!

According to The Cancer Journal for Clinicians even rare cancers are on the rise where 1 in every 5 cancers diagnosed in America is said to be rare cancer. A study called *"the burden of rare cancers in the United States"* published by the cancer journal for clinicians discusses how children and teenagers are 71% more likely to develop a rare cancer type compared to adults, where only 20% were diagnosed in people aged 65 and over. It also said that people diagnosed with a rare cancer type are unlikely to live beyond the 5-year survival rate due to cancer responding poorly to conventional treatments. Based on this study alone you can conclude two things of significance and with some degree of certainty. The first is that you probably won't last 5 years and the second is that they admit that conventional therapies do not work for these cancer types, so why are patients getting them?

Professor Zimmerman himself mentioned in an article that when he was in medical school during the 60s, he was observing a cadaver, a woman who had lung cancer and was told to pay attention because it was so rare that he may never see it again in his practice. Well, I don't need to tell you how common lung cancer is today, so what does that tell you? The age debate for cancer incidence does not explain why children between the ages of 0-14 have leukaemia which accounts for 30% of all cancer in children, brain and spinal cord tumours 26%, Neuroblastoma 6%, Wilms tumour (cancer in the kidneys specific to kids) 5%, Hodgkin's Lymphoma 3%, Non-Hodgkin's Lymphoma 5%, Rhabdomyosarcoma (cancer of the connective tissue between muscle and bone) 3%, Retinoblastoma (cancer of the eye) 2% and bone cancers like osteosarcoma and Ewing sarcoma together make up 3%. These statistics are just for Australia so you can bet your ass that the rest of the world is not missing out.

In 1775 the first cause of cancer was discovered by a British surgeon called Percivall Pott, he had associated the link of scrotum cancer with chimney sweeps during the time. Chimney sweeps were the guys who cleaned all the soot out of the chimney; a master sweep would often take on a young boy who would be trained to climb the chimney and remove the soot. For the children, it was even worse than it sounds as being a chimney sweeps apprentice meant you were essentially an indentured servant. However, it wasn't until the 18th century where things turned to shit and created the foundation of the modern medical problems we have today. This was the time when tobacco was commercialised and the industrial revolution occurred, although technically speaking the industrial revolution started in the mid-17th century and ended in the early 19th century, it wasn't until the early 1800s that cancer escalation began to occur. The industrial revolution caused an epidemic of heavy metal and chemical toxicity and by the time the 1830s had arrived, we were well into our use and abuse of toxic chemicals as demand for these substances grew.

Lawes who produced chemical fertiliser for agriculture rapidly expanded and would soon be one of the largest industries in the world promising higher yields on fewer resources and creating enough food to end the hunger epidemic, which today we know was total bullshit because since that time the hunger epidemic has progressively gotten worse. Corporations that make products with chemicals known to be toxic often use a thing called tobacco science to get them approved. That's because most people in government regulating these industries don't know their ass from a hole in the ground, especially when they are too busy giving themselves a pay raise for stealing our freedoms, destroying the country and disenfranchising its citizens. Some of the worse things that have come from these corporations with the support of government are GMO's, Vaccines, Fluoride, Non-biodegradable Plastics, Chemtrails and ton more which are devastating to human health and biological systems. If you're not familiar with the term tobacco science, it's used to describe a time when we were told that tobacco was not harmful to our health and was even endorsed by your doctor and look how that turned out!

The arguments raised in this book are not new ones and perhaps my unique perspective can help you see what's going on. I feel that most people don't understand what's being said to them and are unwilling to believe that people in positions of power and influence would do this simply because they wouldn't. If you told someone today that smoking is good for you then it's no stretch of the imagination what kind of reaction you would get. God only knows why people cannot see that the advice we are getting today on all of these controversial topics are coming from the same kinds of people, at the same type of authority, with the same mentality, when we were told tobacco and asbestos were safe. Tragically, people still haven't learned, yet they remain quick to judge and slow to change as our problems grow in complexity the longer we ignore them.

So let's take a look at some recent history and explore how well companies and those in authority can lie and deceive a gullible, trusting and ignorant public. After all, billions of dollars have been spent to achieve this very goal and the result is so convincing that companies could put sprinkles on dog shit and sell it as chocolate ice cream and the public wouldn't know the difference.

Tobacco & The Industrial Revolution

Tobacco has always been around even in ancient times and was traditionally chewed or hand-rolled, it wasn't until the invention of the rolling machine by James Bonsack in 1881 did its popularity soar. Nations demand for tobacco even caused wars, the US was a huge producer of tobacco and they used it to finance the American Revolution as well as collateral for the money they borrowed from the French during the war. Many families had owned tobacco plantations and it is considered to be the first crop grown for money, some of the most well-known families in the US growing tobacco was George Washington and Thomas Jefferson. In Australia, you can go to jail longer for growing tobacco than if you were growing marijuana, which is ridiculous considering it's a legal product.

Between 1776 and 1826 the negative health effects of smoking were starting to surface, as technology grew so did the methods of testing its safety and there was a growing concern that it was not as harmless as consumers were led to believe. In 1826 a pure form of nicotine was found and scientists had concluded that it was a dangerous poison. In 1836 Samuel Green of the New England Almanack and Farmer's friend (An Almanack is like a local paper) wrote that tobacco is an insecticide, a poison, a filthy habit and can kill a man, but this had little effect on the popularity that tobacco was gaining.

When the tobacco companies jumped on board they were perpetuating the good health benefits from smoking, even using doctors on advertisements to promote certain brands like Camels and Luckies. Everyone got suckered in, dentists were promoting cigarette filters that wouldn't stain your teeth and even scientists were in the spotlight promoting the use of certain brands. The tobacco industry used the media to make smoking fashionable and soon all the "cool kids" were doing it because they were led to believe it was safe.

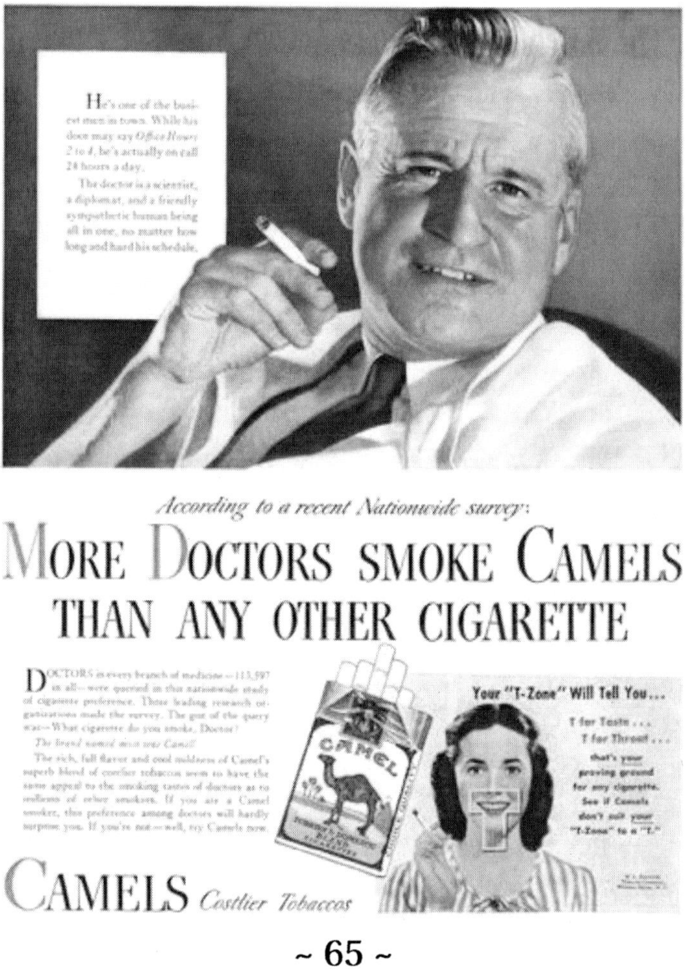

This is a classic example of how ignorant people can be when they blindly believe everything they watch and read without ever questioning, you can see how dangerous this is because today we know exactly what smoking can lead to and its impact on our health.

In the early 1840s, Sir John Lawes founded the chemical fertilizer industry and took out a patent for the creation of superphosphate, a chemical fertiliser, the aim was to boost food production as there was a growing concern about feeding a population which at the time was around 2 billion. The process was done by melting rock and releasing the insoluble minerals like bone and mineral phosphates and converting them into a soluble form like calcium phosphate by reacting with sulphuric or phosphorus acid.

This was the birth of the artificial fertilizer industry and was an important sector of the chemical industry for years to come. Again, we have another connection to agriculture as being a significant contributor to human health and during the industrial revolution, there was an explosion of interest in this industry. Today agriculture is one of the biggest contributors to global pollution and affects just about all biological systems on Earth. The long term effects of chemical fertilizers have yet to be determined, but its use is still allowed even though there is clear evidence that it has hardened our soils by killing beneficial microbes, polluted the land and waterways, contaminated the air and has even made other chemicals more resilient.

This is also the period in time when our use and abuse of Aluminium, Lead, Formaldehyde and Ammonia found their way into the many products that we eat, drink and use daily, all of which can be found in chemical fertilizer and agriculture today.

When you look into the history of these chemicals and heavy metals it's as if a comic was being written, because there is no way on Earth a sane or thinking person would ever allow their use in the products they are found in. All of these substances mentioned are either known to cause cancer or highly suspected to cause cancer in humans and a whole range of other modern diseases that are skyrocketing today. The public has cultivated a mindset of scepticism and doubt and my family at the time were no exception. The whole time my father had cancer he never stopped smoking, he cut back heaps because of his condition but he just couldn't kick the habit, they say it is one of the hardest things to give up which makes sense when you look at all the addictive substances used to make a cigarette.

I remember telling him off about smoking while he was being treated as if chemo and radiation weren't bad enough, but he would always see this as me lecturing him and not the concern for his health. At the time a lecture from me was defined in my family as telling the truth that no one wanted to acknowledge, especially if it meant they had to change or admit they were wrong, the burdens of too much pride. What smokers forget is that non-smokers can smell it a mile away, so when my father sneaked outside I could tell what he was doing even though he lied about it to my face.

Soon after I began to see signs that something was not right in his attitude, even though the oncologist had given him the impression that his condition was treatable. This over-optimistic advice was given by his oncologist and it never included the fact that lung cancer is one of the cancer types with the highest mortality. Knowing my father he would have heard this naive optimism and thought, fuck it! Old habits die hard so why change if I'm going to be alright? Every time I learned something new or shocking about what causes cancer or what made it worse I just had to tell him and my mother whether they wanted to listen or not, but mainly because it contradicted the doctor's advice. I dug deep into our past and found many things that had gained momentum during the industrial revolution which had indicated a significant turning point in not just cancer but all modern disease.

People are always working against their self-interest! Whether its stubbornness, pride, ignorance or just good old fashioned stupidity none of these things are productive in any way whatsoever. It's worse when things go wrong as you predicted and someone you tried to help ignored your message, then they expect you to fix the problem like it was yours too begin with. We have all been there in one way or another. In my family, my parents were acting as if it was ok or fashionable to be oblivious to all these issues as opposed to looking at them as something to learn from. I tried so hard to arm them with what I had learned but they saw my efforts as a hindrance rather than something useful and constructive. I would often hear my parents say things like "The world has gone crazy" especially with all the violent and depressing shit you see on the news every night. The worse thing for me is when you see a child on TV smiling away as they are getting chemo, while the drug company that made it piggybacks the child's suffering to promote their toxic product as some revolutionary breakthrough. Yet despite seeing this news and others like it every night, they remained agnostic to everything I was telling them. I would often try to tell them that a lot of these problems are caused by the things they say I'm lecturing them about, but they would just say no it's not and never explain why. Sometimes I thought, do they just like to argue and be difficult? If so, what a piece of work my family must be! I could have given up and washed my hands of the whole thing as most people would have, but that's not who I am. So I chose to endure the madness of putting up with my parents and their invalid opinions on subjects they never even attempted to understand. Yet the oncologists seemed to possess some kind of supernatural power to persuade them into doing the most ridiculous things that were not even logical.

I realised early on that they had been conditioned like so many others and accepted the doctor's advice as if it were gospel. That's because that's what they were taught and no matter what I said my words would never reach because it contradicted this ideology. I endured as best as I could hoping that I would find a smoking gun that would finally make my parents see the folly of their choice because I knew exactly where this was heading. As I observed this dangerous path my father was on I started to research some of the things that could have contributed to his cancer and was faced with what scientists refer to as "an embarrassment of riches". There was so much evidence in support of toxic products found on the supermarket shelf causing cancer and other diseases that it could only be interpreted as an extreme state of ignorance, or worse, a belief within the scientific community based on little to no facts.

When my parent's told me that the industrial revolution and the products that came from it didn't cause the things I was saying I asked them, how do you know? The only thing you did to understand was to disagree with me, I'm the one who got off their ass and did a bit of research to try and understand because I didn't know. But this was seen as an attempt to start an argument not to prove a point.

Though the tobacco industry certainly had its place, nothing compares to the industrial revolution due to its scale, this is the time when our use and abuse of heavy metals and toxic chemicals established their roots in modern industry and is likely the most responsible period in time for the increase in cancer incidence and modern disease leading to the degradation of human health currently seen today.

It the next part of this book we will explore some of these toxic chemicals and heavy metals such as Aluminium, Formaldehyde, Ammonia, and Lead. Chances are, you have all of them in your home right now and in the last 24hrs used or ate at least one. You must understand what these can do to your health so that you can remove them from your home and make better-informed decisions.

PART II

CHAPTER 4: ALUMINIUM THE SILENT KILLER

On the 15th of October 2010, my father had his left upper lobectomy, this is the removal of his whole left lung including several lymph nodes and was followed by chemotherapy just as the doctor ordered. To make it worse the drug of choice was Cisplatin and Navelbine, two extremely toxic drugs, so much so, that surveys have been done showing that even oncologists wouldn't get Cisplatin for themselves if they had cancer. My father was told that the surgery went well and to be on the safe side they were going to do 4 cycles of chemotherapy, this is standard practice when surgery is an option. He was given the speech oncologists give patients when they think they have beaten someone's cancer, he was told that he was in the clear with no signs of disease in late March 2011 and was due for a review in July that year.

His July check-up came and he passed with flying colours, my family had interpreted this as me being wrong about what I had told them and that the doctors knew what they were doing. But even so, I persisted with learning as much as I could about cancer causation and how it was treated, and soon learned that the doctor's optimism was premature at best. I tried to tell my parents about some of the causes of cancer I had learned and warned my father not to do some of these things because it could make him sick again. It got to the point where I found so many things that can sabotage your immune system and make you chronically sick that they began to wonder if I was paranoid, and even on drugs. Though I had buried myself in alcohol to deal with the mental and emotional anguish the situation caused me they were convinced that something wasn't right with me.

One day my mother was washing my pants after going out with some friends when a white pill had come out of my pocket, they were freaking the hell out! They thought drugs were the cause of all the crazy shit I had been telling them. After 20 minutes of my parents staring at this white pill on the table, my father finally worked up the courage to put it in his mouth and see what it was. Since when has that ever been a good idea?

His face dropped like a dunny seat when he turned and looked at my mother and said, "it's a fucking mint"! It was an Eclipse mint that had come out of my pocket. When they told me about it I said: "FYI drugs usually have a smiley face on them, do I look like I'm smiling"? This proved to me that it wasn't me that was crazy, but it was them for turning a mint into a 20-minute scenario where I was a drug addict!

So here are some of the things I had tried to tell them, at the time I did not know what I know now and this is where you can reap the benefits without going through the painstaking process of trial and error.

Aluminium

This metal is by far one of the most versatile metals we have ever known, yet its effect on human health isn't talked about or even considered in many circles, particularly the industries that produce it. That's because we are doing what we have always done, remaining ignorant to a problem until it is too late to fix. Aluminium makes up 8% of the earth's crust and does not exist in nature in its pure form, it exists as Bauxite, a type of clay or rock. Strangely enough, there is no known biological system on Earth that has a use for aluminium which is almost alien in nature. Yet man has made use of it in just about everything, from planes, trains and automobiles to the foil in your kitchen and everything else in between.

Aluminium even goes back to the Roman days, but it wasn't until 1808 when an English chemist called Humphry Davy thought that aluminium could be produced through electrolytic reduction from alumina (aluminium oxide). Though he never managed to put it in to practice, it turned out he was right and many years later at the beginning of the 20th-century aluminium's use skyrocketed. In 1903 the Wright brothers redesigned the engine of their aeroplane using aluminium parts because the engine was too heavy to get the vehicle off the ground. Around the same time aluminium pots and pans were being commercialised for households everywhere and by 1907 kitchen foil was made by Robert Victor Neher in Switzerland and was even used to wrap the famous chocolate Toblerone.

Some of the other inventions of the 20th century with aluminium at its core were:

- The Empire State Building in 1931
- During WW2 aluminium was used in the manufacture of engines for planes, tanks and automobiles.
- In 1957 the USSR launched the first artificial satellite into orbit using aluminium
- In 1967 Pepsi and Coca-Cola used Aluminium Cans
- In more recent times the Shinkansen (Japanese Bullet train) was made from aluminium. And many more...

There is no shortage of uses with this versatile metal and there is no denying the impact it has had on the modern world, the trouble is that it has also had an impact on our health which has gone largely unnoticed for more than 100 years. What most people don't know is that aluminium and aluminium compounds have found their way into humans and many biological systems through some of the following:

- **Foods** - such as baking powder, self-rising flour, salt, baby formula, coffee creamers, baked goods, processed foods, colouring and caking agents.
- **Drugs** - such as antacids (heartburn), analgesics (pain killers), antidiarrheals and many others.
- **Vaccines** - Hepatitis A and B, Hib, DTaP (diphtheria, tetanus, pertussis), pneumococcal vaccine, Gardasil (HPV), most vaccines use Aluminium Hydroxide an adjuvant.
- **Cosmetics** - Like personal care products such as antiperspirants, deodorants (including salt crystals, made of alum), lotions, sunscreens and additives such as magnesium stearate (used in soaps and shampoos).
- **Aluminium Products** - Foil, cans, juice pouches, tins, water bottles, chemical fertilizer, utensils, pots and pans.
- **Geoengineering** – Nanoparticles of aluminium are used to reflect sunlight off the planet and back into space, apparently this is a countermeasure to combat global warming while it toxifies and acidifies the environment killing many fish and frog species that are sensitive to pH changes.

There is no known safe level of aluminium in the body, yet everyone has it including newborn children. Aluminium is not essential for life and yet despite the debates, it is widely recognized as a neurotoxin which inhibits more than 200 biological functions which are known to adversely affect plants, animals, and humans.

Despite this knowledge, it has contaminated our environment, used in foods, cosmetics, drugs and is done so on the basis that it must be safe because we have always done it. Because aluminium is a neurotoxin it can cause dementia-like symptoms and even Alzheimer's; most people would be shocked to know that dementia and Alzheimer's is a modern disease, of course, these things may have popped up here and there in the past but the scale of it today is extremely alarming.

One thing is for certain, since aluminium's heavy commercialisation between 1903 and 1907, and then its use in vaccines in the 1930s and 1940s Alzheimer's which was first discovered in 1906 has been rapidly increasing ever since. This also coincides with the introduction of aluminium pots and pans into households all over the world and why now it is a subject of global concern. It cannot be a coincidence that during the same period when Aluminium was commercialised by so many different industries that finding it in the home of every person on the planet in one form or another began to increase.

Aluminium has the absolute potential to cause cancer and has strongly been associated with breast cancer due to the use of products containing aluminium and aluminium compounds like those found in antiperspirants and roll-on deodorant. Professor Philippa Darbre at Reading University in the UK noted that in the 1930s and 1940s, 30 % of all breast cancer would appear in the region under the arm where these products were applied. Whereas today nearly 60% of all breast cancer appears in the same region which has been determined by a study taking the fluid from the nipple of women who had breast cancer which showed to have significantly higher levels of aluminium than those who did not have breast cancer.

Professor Darbre's research also showed that not only can aluminium convert a healthy cell into a cancer cell but it also increases the chance of carrying cancer elsewhere in the body by metastasis. Aluminium's role in antiperspirant is to block the sweat glands, however, this is an issue in itself because the whole point of sweating is to cool and detoxify the body by excreting harmful toxins through the skin. This is the body's mechanism for reducing the toxic load in your blood before these toxins can do damage to a vital organ like the brain or heart. By blocking sweating you are allowing the toxins to remain in the body longer and therefore concentrate the toxins in the blood, this puts more stress on the lymph nodes and the immune system as harmful toxins that would normally be flushed out of the body remain there longer leading to chronic diseases like cancer. The thing to bear in mind is that applying deodorant may not give you cancer today or even tomorrow, but you are adding to the bioaccumulation of toxins in your body so it's just a matter of time before something manifests.

Cancers associated with the digestive tract such as mouth, pharynx, oesophagus, stomach, small intestine, large intestine and the anus are also more common in people with aluminium sensitivities. Biochemical researcher H. W. Keens published 2 books back in 1934 and 1937 which discussed the dangers of using aluminium particularly in chemical fertilizers and believed based on his research that it was a primary cause of cancer. Since the 1930s researchers across many fields have become aware that Aluminium can severely impact biological systems and does so in the body by depriving it of essential minerals like sulphur, which is one of the first minerals to be driven out. Why is sulphur so important? It's the third most abundant mineral in the body and is essential for life, aluminium is not. Sulphur makes up vital amino acids used to create protein for cells, tissues, hormones, enzymes and antibodies.

Senior research scientist Stephanie Seneff at MIT University in the US who I was honoured to interview for this book and is considered to be an authority on the issues of Glyphosate which we will discuss later has also found strong links to cancer and autism when Aluminium is combined with Glyphosate. Glyphosate is a chemical compound used in agriculture as an insecticide, herbicide and fungicide. Dr Seneff also noted that the first mineral to go in the body is sulphur and is significantly impacted by the presence of aluminium and the Glyphosate combination. Again we have another link between toxic substances used in agriculture which are used to grow the foods we eat.

Aluminium is also an adjuvant, which is something that's administered to increase immune response and when administered simultaneously with another product say for example peanuts, you can trigger allergic reactions. This was demonstrated to be true in mice by Professor of Pathophysiology and Allergy Researcher, Erika Jensen-Jarolim at the Medical University of Vienna in Austria. However, she went a step further and said that with varying intensity, if we combined aluminium hydroxide with anything in your kitchen we could trigger an allergic reaction. Further studies have demonstrated that aluminium hydroxide is an active ingredient in drugs like heartburn, antacid medication and also vaccines, and when combined with nuts or apple mice in the lab would become allergic to them. So it's no wonder we have all these allergies today, aluminium is also bioaccumulative, dietary aluminium can mostly be flushed through the kidneys, but injectable aluminium from vaccines can take anything between 8 to 15 years before it will leave your body.

Because no safe levels of Aluminium are known this renders the argument useless by health authorities claiming that only a small amount of aluminium enters the body after the application of deodorant, or by injection from a vaccine. This is stupidity on a grand scale and is unbelievably dangerous when authorities tell the public that it is safe. If a substance is bio accumulative and you are regularly exposed to it over an 8 year period, then you don't need to be a genius to realise that you only need a little aluminium to have a huge problem. There is simply no logic to what they claim! If a dog took a shit on your doorstep and you left it there for 8 years it would be gone due to natural decay right? But if a dog took a shit on your doorstep every day for 8 years, what do you think your doorstep would look like? SHIT! So how can it be argued that aluminium and its accumulative nature in the body is any different? Although major health departments like the International Agency for Cancer Research claims that aluminium does not cause cancer, they do recognise that the production of aluminium does, which should have you asking, what is the difference?

A study published in 2009 in the Journal of Inorganic biochemistry by Professor Christopher A Shaw, and Michael S. Petrik called *"Aluminium Hydroxide Injections Lead to Motor Deficits and Motor Neuron Degeneration"* which is exactly what is used in vaccinations today, concluded the following about their safety:

> *Overall, the results reported here mirror previous work that has clearly demonstrated that in both oral and injected forms, can be neurotoxic. Potential toxic mechanisms of action may include enhancement of inflammation (i.e., microgliosis) and the interference with cholinergic projections, reduced glucose utilization, defective phosphorylation-dephosphorylation reactions, altered rate of transmembrane diffusion and selective changes in saturable transport systems in the blood-brain barrier and oxidative damage on cellular processes by the inhibition of the glutathione redox cycle.*

Other researchers that have warned of aluminium and its compounds are Dr Charles Betts of Ohio, who published a book under the auspices of the Anti-Cancer Club of America condemning the use of aluminium. Another is Dr Olds of Philadelphia who stated in a publication that food and water cooked in aluminium vessels caused increased cancer reactions. The University School of Medicine in Belgrade published information showing that drinking water with high aluminium and low fluoride concentration is associated with Alzheimer's risk. This was seen in places like New Guinea, Egypt, Papua Islands and many third world countries where drinking water is contaminated with aluminium and is closely linked to the increase in diseases like amyotrophic lateral sclerosis (ALS) or Parkinson's.

In another study by Philippa D. Darbre, Ferdinando Mannello and Christopher Exley, in the journal of inorganic biochemistry called "*Aluminium and breast cancer: Sources of exposure, tissue measurements and mechanisms of toxicological actions on breast biology*", noted that Aluminium is of historical interest because it has been a suspected carcinogen for more than 100 years. In 1928 a book called 'Aluminium Poisoning' sponsored by the Anti-Cancer Club of America heralded aluminium as "The cause of cancer revealed". However, today Aluminium is not even ranked as a known human carcinogen, officially it is only suspected to be which is why its wide-scale use is still allowed. Aluminium has become so integrated into everyday life that to get rid of it would probably crash the global economy and send us back into the Stone Age.

There is strong evidence that breast cyst fluids are generally higher than blood serum when deodorants are used regularly which is a hidden danger to breastfeeding mothers. Aluminium is also particularly dangerous in premature newborns because their GI tract is underdeveloped. What is most alarming is that if you are using the baby formula on your child as opposed to breastfeeding then the aluminium found in baby formula is even higher than that of breast milk. Aluminium has also been shown to appear in a range of breast structures and not just the cyst fluids, due to aluminium's accumulative nature, the cells most at risk in the body are those that have the slowest turnover like the neurons in the brain.

The human body is well adapted to excreting heavy metals and toxins through the hair, nails, sweat, and urine, but when we are exposed to these toxins daily our bodies become overwhelmed with toxic accumulations whereby disease and disorders are the inevitable results. Some of the health conditions associated with Aluminium are:

Alzheimer's, Autism, Cancer, Osteomalacia, Parkinson's, Acute Appendicitis, Hay Fever, Kidney Disease, Bone Disease, Lung problems, Migraine, Gastric Ulcers, Rheumatism and ductless glands, like the Pituitary, Thyroid, Suprarenal Glands and the sex glands may also get into a disturbed state.

To learn more about aluminium I contacted Christopher Exley Professor of Bioinorganic Chemistry and author of "Aluminium and Alzheimer's disease: The science that describes the link" after seeing him in a documentary called "The Age of Aluminium" which I would highly recommend watching. I asked him if he could tell me about the links between aluminium and cancer which has made up part of this chapter. He told me that there is a huge body of evidence that demonstrates the links between aluminium and many diseases including some cancers, but it is not widely accepted by the mainstream community. His book discusses the research behind the many pathways aluminium can utilize to create cellular damage and also the many diseases that it's suspected of causing. When it comes to aluminium Christopher Exley is one of the world's leading authorities on aluminium toxicity and is someone I would go to if I needed answers.

For any scientist wanting to challenge the science of aluminium's toxicity and the health issues it's associated with, I would highly recommend reading professor Exley's book or getting familiar with his work.

In conclusion, I am not suggesting we undo everything we have done with aluminium, first of all, it would not be practical or realistic. What I hope instead is that people develop a healthy awareness about its toxicity and the potential health dangers it can have, particularly where children are concerned. When I learned of aluminium's toxicity and the million things it is in, I didn't blame my parents for thinking I was paranoid even though what I was saying was the truth. I told them not to get the flu shot or any other type of vaccination, I told them to get rid of their pots and pans for healthier alternatives, I told them what foods and medications had aluminium in it and when I took the aluminium foil out of the kitchen to chuck in the bin I'm sure my parents expected me to make a hat out of it and stick it on my head.

By the time I learned the health dangers of aluminium my father had ignored my advice and was getting chemotherapy to treat his cancer. My mother and I shared taking him to his treatments, but I did the bulk of it because they had a mortgage to pay and her income alone wasn't enough to keep things going. We were under enormous financial stress and the money I had got from Centrelink for caring for him was used to pay bills and put food on the table. It was so fucked up, he was too sick to work but not sick enough to get any kind of financial help from the system he had paid into his whole life. Looking back at things now it's no wonder my words could not reach them, we were all just doing what we had to make it work, so it's no surprise they didn't give two shits about aluminium, there biggest and most immediate concern was keeping a roof over our head. Fortunately, Professor Exley does mention one effective way to help flush aluminium out of your body via the urine, and that is by drinking mineral water high in Silicic acid H4SiO4. This is the bioavailable form of silicon which will bind together and flush it out through the kidneys.

The answers people are looking for are out there! They may not always come in a way we like or accept but they are there. Sometimes, most times, they are staring us in the face and we simply choose to see something else because authorities have told us what the interpretation of them should be. This is a classic example of perception management and is an illusion you must break away from if you are going to take back your health.

CHAPTER 5: AMMONIA! A NEW FOOD GROUP?

Ammonia or Azane is a compound of nitrogen and hydrogen with the formula of NH3, it has that unmistakable pungent smell commonly used in cleaning products and its discovery is said to be as significant as electricity as its uses are numerous.

There is natural ammonia and synthetic ammonia; natural ammonia is released by bacteria, decaying plants, animals and faecal matter, whereas synthetic ammonia is synthesized from natural gas molecules which are reduced to carbon and hydrogen. The hydrogen is then purified and reacted with nitrogen to produce ammonia. Every year man produces nearly as much synthetic ammonia as what naturally occurs, up to 80% of which is used in the chemical fertilizer industry. The discovery of synthetic ammonia was made by German Chemists Fritz Harbor and Carl Bosch on the 13th October 1908, this led to the artificial nitrogen fixation process primarily designed for the chemical fertilizer industry. The process is also known as the Harbor-Bosch process, by taking atmospheric nitrogen and fixing it to the soil using artificial fertilizer they were looking at revolutionising the way food is grown.

It is also said that ammonia has killed as many people as it has helped, although I believe it has done more harm than good considering how we have chosen to use it. It was also used to make Nitro Glycerine, also known as dynamite which the Germans utilised well during WW1.

The negative health effects of ammonia are well known, aside from being blown up by dynamite, it can enter the body by inhalation, touch and ingestion.

When it does the ammonia reacts with the water in your body producing ammonium hydroxide which is highly corrosive and can damage the cells in the lining of your airways. Ammonia is also known to be a potent neurotoxin that can seriously interfere with the nervous system.

A study was done by Dr Aida Adlimoghaddam, at the Division of Neurodegenerative Disorders at St-Boniface Hospital Research Winnipeg in Canada called *"Ammonia as a Potential Neurotoxic Factor in Alzheimer's Disease"*, explains that excessive levels of ammonia have been found in the brains of patients with neurological disorders such as Alzheimer's disease and could be a serious contributing factor. I find it too much of a coincidence that before the 1900s Alzheimer's wasn't even on peoples radar as a disease of concern, it was first discovered by Dr Alois Alzheimer in 1906 as mentioned in the section on aluminium, 2 years before Fritz Harbor utilising a way for the ammonia/nitrogen fixation process used in chemical fertilizer.

From here on out it just snowballs, today in Australia 353,800 people are living with Dementia, which is an umbrella term for neurological disorders like Alzheimer's and it is expected to grow to 400,000 in less than 5 years. Today ammonia is used in the manufacture of dyes, explosives, plastics, drugs, nitric acid, fertilizer and a shit load of other chemicals that contain nitrogen, but the one that scares me the most is that 70% of all supermarket ground beef has ammonia in it. Health authorities tell us that ammonia is used to kill E.coli which is why it's in ground beef, that sounds great except the human body is estimated to have 39 trillion bacteria which it is also affecting and they don't take into account what the health impact is.

Jamie Oliver even did a short YouTube video demonstrating how ammonia is used in ground beef to raise awareness about what people are really eating and is worth a watch if you're after a visual demonstration.

Authorities that allow chemicals like ammonia to exist in our food like to explain away the problem by saying things like...

"It's in low concentrations so it's not harmful", or

"We have been using it for years and you're the first to bring it to our attention", and my favourite...

"There are no scientific studies to prove it's harmful to people"

When in reality there exists dozens and sometimes hundreds of scientific studies that they have chosen to ignore so when they get questioned about it they can honestly say that they have never seen it. The concentration of a chemical in a product is usually a central point of debate for authorities but even so, I seriously doubt that anyone would want even a fraction of ammonia in their food when it's also used in commercial cleaning products, plastics, explosives, fertilizers and domestic cleaners. Parents are often told to lock cupboard doors so children don't ingest chemicals from under the sink but many of these chemicals we are told to keep out of reach with children are ending up in our food anyway.

Here's a wild thought, how about manufacturers and distributors of these products find better and safer practices that do not require the use of ammonia, God forbid we should support local producers who can get fresh organic products to our door without the use of such chemicals for the sake of extending shelf life. Many studies have been done on the environmental impact of ammonia, particularly on aquaculture as many species appear to be extremely sensitive to the chemical. The average concentration of ammonia reported at hazardous waste sites range between 1ppm to 1,000 ppm, some samples in the soil are as high as 3,000ppm and in water samples 16 ppm. Yet it only takes 0.02 ppm to be considered potentially harmful and even kills fish, so it's no wonder you get mass fish deaths popping up all over the world especially in the US, although over the last few years Australia has also had its fair share.

If ammonia is so great then why does it say on the bottle that if you see symptoms of ammonia poisoning, not like most people know what they are, to contact your local poison control centre? Pfitzer the pharmaceutical company released a study that tells of ammonia's role in cancer and how it acts as a diffusible signal that triggers autophagy, meaning that when the cancer cells are put under stress by chemotherapeutic agents, the ammonia tells the neighbouring cancer cells to prepare for an attack by the immune system making them more resistant to treatment and harder to kill. This is why meat unless it is organic or wild-caught, are excluded from the cancer recovery diet, and even then it could pose problems depending on your cancer type. Beef and other red meats have been strongly associated with causing colorectal cancer and can increase your risk of other cancers as well. A study by the Department of Preventive Medicine in the Kyoto Prefectural University of Medicine in Japan called *"Effect of ammonia on cell-cycle progression of human gastric cancer cells"* suggested that ammonia and ammonia chloride inhibit the growth of gastric cells during the S-phase of the cell cycle.

The S-phase of the cell cycle is where the cell produces two similar daughter cells and also when DNA replication occurs, well this is a big problem because as we learned earlier if the DNA is damaged during replication process then it can become cancerous, and since ammonia is in most beef products this is why it is strongly suspected of causing colorectal cancer. As mentioned earlier natural ammonia is produced by decaying matter, but it is also produced as a by-product of the cell cycle, in another study by the Department of Cell Biology at Harvard Medical School in Boston Called *"Metabolic recycling of ammonia via glutamate dehydrogenase support breast cancer biomass"* shows that the recycling of ammonia accelerated the proliferation of cells in breast cancer. So just imagine what elevated levels of ammonia must be doing when you consume meat products treated with this chemical.

Ammonia is but one chemical among 100's that could be contributing to the cancer epidemic and what I believe to be the ever-growing feedback loop mentioned earlier. The fact that more studies haven't been done on ammonia despite its known toxic side effects and its widespread use is extremely alarming. Yet the official position of health authorities remain that ammonia in cleaning products is poisonous as mentioned on the bottle, but when it's used in meat products at the deli it is not, which makes no fucking sense at all!

After I told my parents about ammonia and what it can do to people with cancer they found it difficult to accept and that's because they had grown up as most Australians do, where every meal as a meat meal. Humans can be so deranged in there logic, you can warn them of dangerous chemicals and heavy metals but when they find it in their favourite product they try and justify its continued use and still want to be healthy? This is willful ignorance on an epic scale and is the essence of real evil in our world today.

CHAPTER 6: CH2O THE KNOWN HUMAN CARCINOGEN

Formaldehyde is one of the oldest known chemicals in the world and it is estimated that man uses more than 20 million tons each year. Formaldehyde is a clear, water-white, slightly acidic, gas or liquid; it is a naturally occurring chemical compound made up of carbon, hydrogen and oxygen and was formally discovered in 1868 by August Wilhelm von Hofmann a professor of chemistry and director of the laboratory of the University of Berlin.

Formaldehyde began in Germany and by the 1900s gained popularity when the United States, France and Belgium began to use it in the medical industry. Approximately 1.5 ounces of formaldehyde is produced each day by the body due to its normal metabolic functions, it is broken down quickly in the water of your body where 37% of it stays in the aqueous solution from formalin a water-soluble form of formaldehyde.

Formaldehyde is another useful albeit dangerous chemical to have emerged from the industrial revolution. Today formaldehyde is used in the manufacturing process of many products such as glues and adhesives, plastics, rubber, fabrics, clothing, paper, particleboard, floor coverings like carpet, insulation, timber panelling, plywood, cosmetics and other personal care products like lotions, shampoos, sunscreens, soap, body wash, toothpaste, baby wipes, bubble bath, heaps of cleaning products, fuels and fuel additives (Petroleum-based), paints and paint additives, electronic products, vaccines, medications, water treatment products, it even has minor uses in agriculture.

If you see any of these names on any product you have bought, it is likely a compound of formaldehyde:

Formalin, Methanal, Oxymethylene, Urea, 1,3-Dioxetane, Quaternium 15, Methyl aldehyde, Methylene Oxide, Formic Aldehyde, Oxomethane Formalin and Phenol-Formaldehyde.

Bear in mind that no company will disclose the use of Formaldehyde on a product label and that's because it is also a known human carcinogen, instead, they have all the other fancy names that you cannot pronounce which are compounds or derivatives of this cancer-causing chemical.

Formaldehyde is known to cause cancer particularly of the nasopharynx and sinus but it can also cause leukaemia. Studies have shown statistically relevant information associating formaldehyde with pancreatic, brain and lung cancer, though it is generally accepted that more research needs to be done. Formaldehyde has been linked to allergies and asthma in children and can even cross the placenta and enter the fetal tissues. It has even been shown to penetrate the blood-brain barrier and impact the liver. Formaldehyde is particularly toxic when inhaled as a gas, which explains the torrent of respiratory issues people can get from exposure, but what about when your doctor gives it to you as a treatment or drug? In the traditional sense formaldehyde was used to embalm corpses for medical examinations, but today we use it for a whole range of other medical issues.

It is used to dry the skin before and after the removal of warts, it's used to get rid of athlete's foot, it's in cough drops, skin disinfectants, mouthwashes, spermicide creams, used to sterilize cysts before surgery and is even used in root canals. Vets have used it in the treatment of footrot in cattle and it's in a whole range of parasite medications, antiseptics, fumigant's and is used to treat conditions like tympany, diarrhoea, mastitis, pneumonia and internal bleeding.

The Environmental Protection Agency formally listed Formaldehyde as a human carcinogen in 1987, yet despite this, we still use it in many products today like scented candles, though the candles themselves don't contain formaldehyde the citric scented candles in particular which have limestone added to them mutates into formaldehyde when it is burned and has contact with the air. A study was conducted by Professor Alastair Lewis of the National Centre for Atmospheric Science at the University of York said that the levels of Formaldehyde are 100 times more than previously thought and are higher than those in medical students exposed to dead bodies where formaldehyde was used to preserve them.

Some of the symptoms of exposure to formaldehyde are nosebleeds, sore throats, coughs and stinging eyes, so the next time you burn a scented candle if you get any of these symptoms to stop immediately and open a window to air out the home. Alternatively, find more natural ways to scent the home like using organic oils in aromatherapy which can be very beneficial to cancer recovery for stress relief. Professor Lewis also recommends that household plants such as English ivy, geraniums, lavender and many ferns are the best to remove Formaldehyde from the air along with other toxic airborne chemicals, so consider getting some of these for the home if you want to improve your air quality.

In 1978 researchers found in a carcinogenic study on formaldehyde and rats over 2 years that after 18 months 36 of the rats had developed nasal cancers at 14.3 ppm, which was a rare type of cancer in rats and was a cause for immediate concern, other studies followed and by 1987 it was determined to be a known human carcinogen. Even though very little was understood at the time about the mode of action formaldehyde has in cancer development, today we have the studies that show more conclusive results of its effects. Despite the research that warns of its carcinogenic potential we have done nothing to remove or replace it in the manufacture of products which we are told poses no harm to our health because it's in relatively small amounts.

Earlier I mentioned what the ramifications would be if the anti-cancer establishment endorsed the use of a cancer-causing product, well formaldehyde is the next best thing. If you go on to the Cancer Councils website they clearly say that formaldehyde possesses no serious risk to the general public and that even though it is in everyone's home only those with extreme sensitivities may have reactions to it. This is one of the most unscientific statements I have ever heard, no two people are the same so of course, some people are going to be more affected than others, that said, even those that don't show sensitivities immediately doesn't mean it hasn't affected them.

The International Agency for Research on Cancer (IARC) has classified formaldehyde as Group 1, which is defined as carcinogenic to humans, officially it's still allowed to be used in small amounts. So there you have it!

The authorities admit that they are allowing people to be exposed to a known human carcinogen, what more proof do you want? Formaldehyde is used in shit you wouldn't believe, and on the subject of shit, I should probably mention that it has also been found in toilet paper where the thicker and more bleached the toilet paper is, the higher the concentration of irritant chemicals. Formaldehyde is also used in facial tissues, paper towel, toilet paper and other paper products to achieve certain characteristics like wet strength, shininess and absorbability where it was found that the thicker and more expensive the product is the more formaldehyde was present. In a study called *"Chronic vulvar irritation: Could toilet paper be the culprit?"* by Dr Baukje Miedema at the Dalhousie University Family Medicine Teaching Unit at the Dr Everett Chalmers Regional Hospital found some interesting things about the humble dunny roll, she concluded the following in her study:

There are more than 100 000 chemicals used in commercial products. Few have been tested for possible risks to health, yet those risks can be considerable. We postulated that there must be a chemical that remains in the bleached toilet paper that acts as an irritant or allergen. We contacted several toilet paper manufacturers but were unable to obtain a list of the chemicals used to produce toilet paper. All manufacturers refused to provide consumer information, claiming proprietary rights to trade secrets.

As clinicians, we suggest that when a woman presents to her family physician with chronic vulvar problems, the usual standard of care be applied. However, if all test results are negative and no cause can be determined, the patient should be advised to use unbleached toilet paper or minimally processed toilet paper to see if her symptoms abate. This is an easy, low-cost, and non-invasive suggestion that might solve the patient's problem. Further, as a result of this case study, we believe that it is crucial that the manufacturers of toilet paper and other personal hygiene products and household goods be required to reveal all ingredients and chemicals in their products.

So basically, it's legal for companies to manufacture a product using cancer-causing chemicals and they can protect themselves using the trade secret excuse under intellectual property law. Since when is it legal to poison consumers and not disclose ingredients? If you or I did this we would be drawn and quartered by authorities! I don't think I'm alone in saying that when I park my breakfast in the morning and go to wipe my ass, I shouldn't have to think if my fucking toilet roll is poisoning me! And if there are any odd sensations back there after doing so you can bet your ass that I am not going to be quiet about it! So the next time you go to the toilet and experience any tingling sensations just remember that it might not be the Indian or Mexican you had the other night, it could be something far more sinister.

The government has also used this tactic under intellectual property law to avoid answering many legitimate and damaging questions. If you submit a freedom of information request to any government department legally they have to reply, but many government agencies have used companies for their research so when people such as myself send an FOI request then as a private company they can legally refuse to answer claiming it's to protect the secrets of their product. This is how so many legitimate questions continued to go unanswered and why manipulation of laws and regulations allow them to legally get away with it.

Formaldehyde is used in so many products that it further validates the daily burdening of the human body exposed to chemicals resulting in chronic diseases. Even brand new clothes at your favourite retailer are exposing you to formaldehyde which is used to keep the creases out of clothing, so it just goes to show how all of these little things that are hiding in plain sight are gradually adding up to the chronic diseases we are seeing today.

CHAPTER 7: LEATHAL LEAD

Lead is another one of those metals that goes back to ancient times and was even named the father of all metals. Lead has been used everywhere particularly by the Romans which is where chemical symbol Pb comes from. The Latin word for lead which is "Plumbum" is where the word plumber comes from, which is a maker of lead pipes. Lead was used all over Rome even in the famous Aqua Duct, yet surprisingly even back then the Romans knew about leads toxicity. Despite this awareness, the Romans used it in pipes to carry water which they drank and bathed in regularly. They also boiled wine in led vessels to create lead acetate which is sweet to the taste, this was done to improve the palatability of the wine which says a lot about the taste of their wine.

Some historians believe that the Romans extensive use of this toxic metal may have even led to the fall of the Roman Empire, but nothing is conclusive. Before lead is made it is locked up in Galena, a bluish, grey, or black mineral of metallic appearance, which is approximately 87% lead and 13% sulphide. The radioactive element Uranium and a couple of other radioactive elements actually decay into lead and is used in geology to date the earth; this process is also where the majority of the earth's lead comes from. Before 2004, Australia was the largest producer of lead in the world which have since been overtaken by China. Historically speaking lead has had some wonderful uses, due to leads high-density lead aprons were used to shield doctors using equipment with a high radiation output like X-rays and CT scans.

But by far the best and most useful inventions for lead was the lead-acid battery which was used in motor vehicles and tones of other electronics all over the world. Approximately 85% of the worlds lead is used to make batteries where China is the largest manufacturer. However, the lead-acid battery for your car is not made of pure lead, it's made of recycled lead, a lead alloy, which is the reason why your car battery dies after a year or so, try to keep in mind that we are talking about big companies here so there is no money in producing a battery that lasts forever. Just like there is no money in healing the sick, the term for this is called "Planned Obsolescence" it means that things are designed with a lifespan to keep people consuming. Batteries with 99.99% pure lead are those used in hospitals as backups for blackouts, so a better battery does exist. A great documentary to watch on YouTube is called the "Light Bulb Conspiracy", in a certain fire station in the US they celebrate the 110th birthday of the light globe in their fire station proving that things can be built to last.

Lead also found its way into household paints which was noted for its durability; the problem was kids being kids would put paint flakes riddled with lead into their mouth which as we know from the Romans was sweet to the taste. At one stage even baby cribs were painted with lead-based paints which resulted in infant illness and death. Due to the increase in incidence in 1922 the League of Nations during WW1 which was made up of 63 countries including Australia, banned the use of lead-based paint due to its known toxicity, but I guess Australia didn't get that memo because we continued to use it for many years after.

Lead-based paint is just as toxic today as it was back then and if you live in Australia and your house was built before 1970 it's worth getting your house and soil tested for lead exposure as you will soon learn why.

From 1970 onwards lead in paint has been gradually phased out and I believe that the acceptable level now is 0.1% according to the Department of the Environment and Energy. Lead also found its way into the fuel of every motorist in the form of Tetra-ethyl lead (CH3CH2)4Pb and truly goes down in history as one of the greatest human health and environmental fuck-ups of all time. Lead was added to fuel for its anti-knock properties which increased an engine's performance and made the vehicle run quieter. Coincidently in 1922 when the League of Nations banned lead-based paint around the same time it was starting to be used in fuel and many countries including America and Australia ignored the growing concerns of lead's toxicity.

In 1921 Charles F Kettering, vice president for research at General Motors and his chief research assistant Thomas A Midgely tested tetra-ethyl lead in gasoline for the first time while the subsidiaries of Standard Oil and Du Pont would produce the product at their growing refineries. The product tetra-ethyl lead was viciously defended by the group claiming that there was no alternative and was the only thing that could increase an engine's performance while maintaining the desired anti-knock properties leaded fuel provided. However, one alternative that was being researched at the time was a blend of alcohol and benzene, benzene is another known human carcinogen and in my opinion, could have produced side effects just as bad as lead. Researchers said that the alcohol and benzene blend was more reliable than tetra-ethyl lead, but the group not straying from what they specialized in combined with spending considerable time and money did not want to replace it with something new.

Between 1923 and 1925 Thomas A Midgely suffered lead poisoning due to his close involvement with the product, members of his team had also become very ill due to their exposure. However, despite controversial debates on public health Midgely assured that it would not be a health concern to the public and soon after it was in the vehicle of every motorist. A few years earlier in 1906 Standard Oil the US's largest refiner who was later producing tetra-ethyl lead was charged with the monopolising of the oil industry so these guys were dodgy as to being with. The court was completely overwhelmed with testimony and bombarded with enormous amounts of evidence for market manipulation, industrial spying, price-cutting and much more. Yet despite the overwhelming evidence demonstrated in court the judges just dismissed all of the evidence and on May 15, 1911, Standard Oil was ordered by the courts to be dissolved which essentially became 20 separate companies all from the same parent company which adopted the same philosophy of controlling the market.

The 5 major US companies that emerged from the split was Mobile, Exxon, Texaco, Chevron and Gulf which had partnered with 2 international companies BP and Shell, together they are known as the 7 sisters, which today are descendants of Standard Oil. The court's ruling did nothing to change the way these subsidiary companies do business or even become more competitive, nor did it punish the executives who were responsible for these unlawful acts.

They were told that whatever the percentage of shares they held in the trust they owned, they would get the same percentage in the subsidiary companies. A year or 2 later share prices had more than doubled for the subsidiaries and so the dissolving of Standard Oil turned out to be more profitable doubling the CEO's salaries who were responsible in the first place. The largest shareholder of the group was John D Rockefeller, the very same John D Rockefeller who financed the pharmaceutical industry that we currently know today.

So what does this have to do with lead in fuel? Well on September the 4th, 1946 a patent was registered by Harold E Crozier and Albert G H Yanderpole for an anti-knock or detonation dampening device using water, not lead, which Shell Oil had covered up. So, in essence, the human health and environmental hazard lead caused and still does to this day could have been avoided if it wasn't for a group of greedy lying assholes trying to line their pocket at everyone's expense. It has been said that Thomas A Midgely and the use of lead in fuel is responsible for more damage to Earth's atmosphere than any other single organism that has ever lived. At least 235,000 tons of lead-based emissions from motor vehicles were released into the environment in Australia all of which are still toxic today.

So why is lead so toxic? It is well known that lead is a neurotoxin and like aluminium and many other heavy metals it is also bioaccumulative, there are no safe levels of lead in the human body and towns that have been close to lead mining, or smelting know all about the dangers of lead.

Broken Hill in NSW Australia is also where Mining Company BHP was founded, that's why it's called Broken Hill Proprietary

Company Limited (BHP) founded back in 1885. BHP's activities in Broken Hill have turned the entire town into a toxic hazard that no one knows how's to clean up, that's because there is no uniform way on how to handle widespread contamination of lead, yet to this day they continue to spread it.

At least 1/5th of the town's children currently have lead levels well over the Australian benchmark which is 10 micrograms/dc, yet the natural level of lead in pre-industrial humans is 0.016 microgram/dc, that's 625 times the natural levels. 10 micrograms/dc, is enough to drop a child's IQ by 7 points, that enormous! Professor Kim Dietrich who conducted the largest study in the world on lead and crime rates said that he would kill for an increase in 7 IQ points it's that significant.

When lead enters the bloodstream it is excreted in urine and bile at a clearance rate of 1 to 3 mL/min, with a half-life of approximately 30 days. The remaining lead binds to red blood cells and gets deposited into soft tissues which eventually get deposited in the bone. The body mistakes lead for calcium and that's because they both compete for the same protein which helps the nervous system to function, unlike lead, calcium is essential for healthy brain function. Lead deposited in the bone has a half-life range of 20-30 years which is why you only need to be exposed to a small amount regularly to have a huge impact on your health. When your body needs calcium the lead in your bones is released and is then able to travel anywhere in the body including the brain. Lead in the brain damages nerves and the neuro system and if you are pregnant it will not only go to the brain of the mother but can cross the placenta and affect the unborn child as well. It has even been shown in studies that newborn babies often have a blood lead level similar to the mother. Although lead is harmful to both children and adults children absorb lead twice as fast and those most at risk are children, pregnant woman and those who may already have an illness. It has also been shown that leads toxicity is increased in people due to poor nutrition, deficiencies in calcium, iron, and zinc as well as other nutritional factors.

Lead is also known for its ability to change human behaviour, particularly an increase in violence and criminal behaviour. Consistent neuropsychological research over the years has revealed that lead exposure can result in declines in intelligence, memory, processing speed, comprehension and reading, visuospatial skills, motor skills and to a probable lesser extent, executive skills.

Some of the signs of lead poisoning in adults are:

Miscarriages, Premature Births, Low Birth Weight, Brain damage, Decreased Mental Abilities, Learning Difficulties, Personality Changes, Memory & Coordination Problems, Hearing & Vision Impairments, Muscle & Joint Pain, Reproductive Problems (Men and Women), Headaches, Neuropathy, Weakness, Foot & Wrist Drop, Stomach Aches, and Cancers of the Kidney, Brain and Lung.

Those in children are:

Learning Difficulties as well as Irritability, Coma and Death, Fatigue, Lower IQ, Lack of Attentiveness, Encephalopathy (A disease where the brains function is impaired by a toxin), Nausea, Slowed Growth, Hyperactivity, Vomiting, Gaiting

Disturbances, Seizures, and also Cancers of the Kidney, Brain and Lung.

In both children and adults, pale skin due to anaemia could be an early sign because lead interferes with the production of haemoglobin. Government agencies and the industries that produce lead and lead compounds are significantly playing down the role lead plays in cancer causation and human health. According to the American Cancer Society inorganic lead is classed as a 2A carcinogen, which is defined as probably carcinogenic to humans, and only 2 classes away from known carcinogens like Formaldehyde, Mercury, Benzene, Plutonium. What I find odd is that the National Toxicology Program which is a part of the U.S Department of Health and Human Services has a report on carcinogens associated with lead and lead compounds which were first listed in 2004, CAS No. 7439-92-1 (Lead). On the first page under "Cancer Studies in Humans" it says, lead exposure has been associated with increased risk of lung, stomach, and urinary bladder cancer in diverse human populations and concluded the following:

Carcinogenicity was observed in studies with inorganic lead compounds, both soluble (lead acetate and lead subacetate) and insoluble (lead phosphate, lead chromate), and with tetraethyl lead (an organic lead compound that used to be in Gasoline). Lead caused cancer in rats and/or mice exposed orally, by injection, or perinatally (via the placenta or lactation).

Benign and malignant kidney tumours (adenoma, carcinoma, and adenocarcinoma) were most frequently associated with lead exposure, and tumours of the brain, hematopoietic system, and lung were reported in some studies (IARC 1980, 1987).

The report also mentions that after pregnant mice were given lead acetate in their drinking water from day 12 to four weeks postpartum, the offspring showed dose-related increase's in proliferative lesions of the kidneys including atypical hyperplasia, adenoma, and adenocarcinoma.

What makes lead such a dangerous and alarming metal is the seemingly harmless products we find it in, for example, a study by Researcher Sa Liu, S. Katharine Hammond, and Ann Rojas-Cheatham called *"Concentrations and Potential Health Risks of Metals in Lip Products"* concluded that heavy metal toxicity in lipstick products are a serious concern for woman's health. 32 lip products were taking from 7 distant companies which included 8 lipsticks and 24 lip glosses ranging in price from $5.59 - $24 and found lead in 75% of them above the national safety standard set out by the FDA of 0.01%. The study also concluded that other toxic heavy metals like Manganese (Mn), Titanium (TI) and Aluminium (Al) were found in all products and at the highest levels.

Lead can be found in cosmetics, fishing sinkers, the water supply, trace elements of Arsenic (As), Cadmium (Cd) and Lead (Pb) were found in chemical fertilisers used in agriculture, but also in canned food and chocolate, it's also in the spice turmeric in the form of lead chromate. Lead chromate in turmeric I found to be a shock because it doesn't need to be there, out of all the things you could give a recovering cancer patient turmeric is at the top of the list, there is a ton of research into the positive health benefits of turmeric especially for improving memory, reducing inflammation and also its anti-cancer properties. It's interesting to me that lead chromate is yellow like turmeric, looks and feels like turmeric, and is sweet to the taste of turmeric. Call it a conspiracy theory if you like but there are too many similarities between the two for it to be just coincidence, so make up your own mind.

On Pub Chem which is part of the National Institute of Health, this is what they say about lead chromate:

Lead chromate is highly corrosive and is a strong oxidizing agent. This substance is used in printing books and to color vinyl, rubber, and paper. Lead chromate primarily affects the lungs causing shortness of breath, bronchitis, pneumonia, and asthma but can also affect the gastrointestinal tract, liver, kidneys and immune system. This substance is a known human carcinogen and is associated with an increased risk of developing lung cancer and cancer of the sinonasal cavity.

This is the exact reason why 6 brands of turmeric were recalled because lead chromate should not be in food PERIOD! Call me old fashioned, but if you define something as probably carcinogenic to humans but you don't know 100%, you don't put something you think might cause cancer in the food people buying and say let's see what happens, the general public is not a testing ground for incompetence, greed or stupidity.

Lead and lead compounds to avoid are Lead Chromate, Lead Acetate & Sub Acetate, Lead Phosphate and Tetraethyl lead.

The cancer types associated with lead and lead compounds are Lung Cancer, Stomach Cancer, Urinary-Bladder Cancer, Brain Cancer (Gliomas), benign and malignant Kidney tumours, and Cancer of the Sinonasal Cavity.

Common products with lead and lead compounds are:

Paints, Pigments, and other artists' supplies, Lead Crystal, Protective/Decorative Coatings, Jewellery, Decorative Figurines, Fastenings and trim on clothing, Fishing Sinkers and Jigs, stained glass windows and doors, Batteries, Traditional cosmetics – Lipstick, Lotions, Toothpaste, Pencils, and even Tap water.

Better alternatives have always existed and in many ways, the suppression of better technologies with water-based fuel systems is no different to that of alternative cancer treatments today.

In the US in 1986 Stan Meyer made a fuel cell that could run on water, there was enormous interest in this and was even covered by the media all over the country. The Pentagon was extremely interested in the design because it could run on freshwater, saltwater, lake water and snow, and Stan said that it would cost roughly $1,500 and that it doesn't require any maintenance. He was even offered a billion dollars by oil-producing companies for the design but refused to sell. The day after he made the deal with the Pentagon Stan was murdered, on the day of his murder Stan was out the front doing something until his brother Stephen Meyer heard his brother yell in distress, he ran outside shouting what's wrong to Stan and all Stan could say before he died was "They poisoned me"...

Other Inventors who developed fuel-less cars that could run on water were Edwin Gray, John Robert Fish, and Charles Nelson Pogue, all papers and inventions from these people have been actively suppressed. The following quote is from Stan Meyer in 1997.

We can demonstrate the technology. We can say it's here, but in actuality, it will not be Stan Meyers to bring it in. It will be either you or I, the guy down the street, who will come together to bring it in. Otherwise, I do not believe an alternate energy source, whether water fuel cell or other, would ever come in. It's going to have to be mandated by the people to try to reverse the environmental problems, the environmental damage, that's actually occurring

The history of lead and cancer is but one link in the chain of why we have so much illness in the modern age, again it's not like better options weren't available it's that they simply weren't profitable. People often struggle with the idea that big corporations wouldn't do this and I always say, you wouldn't do this to people, they would. I don't know why some people have such a difficult time accepting that not everyone subscribes to the same logic as them. I'm not one for quoting Madonna but I'm a material girl in a material world seems to be the message put out there buy these globalist corporations to keep people consuming, even at the expense of their health.

Before you make some careless assumption about what you think people are capable of, maybe you should look into our history, you know Hitler, Napoleon, Stalin, Pol Pot, Ted Bunday, James Warren Jones, our history is loaded with psycho's who get off on this shit. Many of the worlds CEO's are said to be sociopaths and that's because they are prepared to do the things that the rest of us wouldn't. History has seen plenty of people like this and the world turns to shit fast when these kinds of people assume positions of authority, power and influence.

As a final caution on heavy metal and chemical toxicity, it's important to mention the common reoccurring theme with these types of substances and that is their ability to go under your radar. In many cases, you cannot see, taste, touch or smell these hidden dangers in the everyday products we use and that is why your general awareness needs to improve.

We will conclude this part of the book with this example. Here is a beautiful frog, it's called Dendrobatidae, also known as the poison dart frog of the Amazon and is so poisonous that one touch of its skin could kill as many as 20 adult men and 10,000 mice.

The products we use every day and assume are safe are much like this frog. It is appealing to the eye, you may want to touch it, or even eat if you got hungry enough, but doing so would mean certain death, you're beliefs or perspective on this fact is irrelevant!

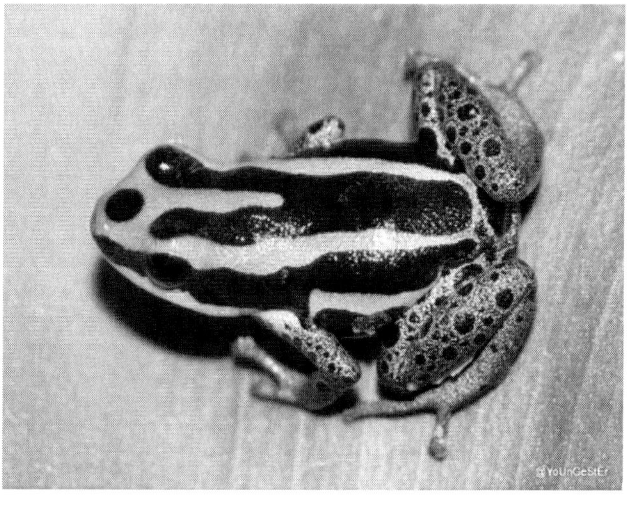

PART III

CHAPTER 8: GMO's HAVE GOT TO GO!

In early 2012 my life had done a 180-degree turn, I was working in insurance as an account manager and I'm not joking when I say that insurance is where dreams go to die. I had found out that my best friend Carlo had killed himself, he hung himself in a tree at a reserve near his mother's house, she had already lost her husband in a car accident many years earlier and now her son and my best friend was gone, I still can't imagine how she must have felt losing her whole family like that.

On the 14th of April 2012, Carlos funeral was held and coincidently it was also my fathers birthday. I wondered if he was being shown a sign and that if he didn't listen to his body and stop taking his health for granted that a decision would be made for him, one that he would not return from. When I saw Carlos mother at the funeral I thought she was being very cold, until I realised that she was on enough Valium to drop a horse, if she wasn't then I doubt she would have kept it together. Despite our differences, his loss had affected me and began to show in my work as I was soon fired from my crappy little insurance job. Everything spiralled out of control, the rego on my car expired so I had no car, I had no job, no money to pay for bills, my girlfriend left me for reasons not worth mentioning, and to top it all off my father had developed a persistent cough making me fear the worse.

After multiple CT scans and biopsies in the lung, it was a bronchoscopy that confirmed the cause of my father's cough. A bronchoscopy is where they put a camera in the lung to see what is going on, and a Bronchoalveolar lavage (BAL) is where they squirt fluid into the lung and collect it to test for infectious diseases.

These tests had found grown Penicillium marneffei in the lung, which is now called Talaromyces marneffei and is in the top 10 most feared fungus in the world. A month of antifungal medication proved useless and when it was positively identified the medication he needed had to come from overseas because it was so rare that it just isn't seen in Australia. He was probed with questions from the doctor about travelling to Aisa because that is where it is found. But because he was home all the time they completely excluded the possibility that his treatment had sabotaged his immune system allowing him to pick up what was floating around in the hospital where he was being treated.

On a routine check-up in late August that year, our fears were confirmed, his cancer had returned and in the oncologists own words it was Small Cell Lung cancer, which is a more aggressive type of lung cancer. With his previous treatment, the CT scans the biopsies plus the fungal infection it was no wonder this was the result, yet my father proceeded with chemotherapy and radiation just as the doctor ordered. The chemo drug of choice this time was Carboplatin and Etoposide another two extremely toxic drugs including radiation on his chest and his head. The disturbing part about this is that the long term side effects were not even discussed with my parents before they committed him to this insanity! And before I knew it I was back in the thick of it dealing with doctors bullshit and my parent's ignorance even after I had told them this could happen.

I am not bullshitting you when I say that I felt as if I had been denied everything good in this world and It was by far my lowest point, or at least I thought at the time. The stress of not knowing whether he would live or die and the ongoing financial pressure was maddening and I honestly don't know how I endured it.

After more research, I had told my father that this time things have to be different and that I would ask the oncologist 3 questions to prove that they cannot help you to overcome this disease. Reluctant to agree I think he did in the end just to stop me from going on about it. I drove him to Box Hill hospital for his appointment and sat in the waiting room rehearsing what I had learned and eager to put it in to practice. After waiting 30mins or so it was time to see the oncologist, she seemed nice and friendly but I wasn't going to let that deter me. I'd rather a doctor is who an arrogant egomaniac who knows what they are doing than someone who is nice and has no clue, so I asked her directly these 3 questions…

- What alternatives are there to surgery, chemotherapy, and radiation?
- What is the name of the chemo drugs you're recommending and what are the full side effects?
- If you or a family member was in the same position as my father would you still be recommending the exact same treatment?

To the first question she answered without hesitation, there are no other treatments, but I knew that gene therapy and immune therapy is something mainstream she could have offered him especially for lung cancer, but she never brought it up. To the second question, she said there could be some appetite loss, hair loss, burning sensations, possible nausea and some other short-term side effects.

The more serious long term side effects were NOT mentioned, some of them are secondary cancers, infertility and even death. This is why you want to leave with a list in your hand so you can fact check this at home before you commit to this type of treatment, and if the side effects don't match what you have been told, then confront them on it and demand an explanation, after all, you are the one that has to take it, not them! The third answer she gave was the most surprising because she did her best to avoid answering it by deflecting the question the way a politician does when you have caught them in a lie.

I was positive that after seeing her response to my questions that my father would reconsider or at least start to question if they knew what they were doing, but he continued with the treatment like nothing important just happened. I began to realize that maybe my father didn't want to survive his cancer which at the time seemed like a crazy thought, but as time passed I realised that maybe there was something to this.

I refused to accept defeat and play the role of the grieving victim, I was determined to change what I knew was wrong, and I refused to let the emotional burden of his disease tear my family apart as everyone blindly followed his doctor's advice. I found it more constructive to be angry with everyone than give in to despair, which gave me the drive and motivation I needed to research more on cancer and the controversy surrounding it. Sometimes you don't know what you are looking for until you ask the right question. When I did, I realized that there were potentially hundreds of things causing cancer to everyday people, the difficult part was connecting the dots until I could see a picture.

In this part of the book, we are going to look at what I believe are some of the biggest contributors to cancer causation and modern disease. So far we have covered the toxicity of some chemicals and heavy metals so we can honestly say that if they are present in any food, water or product we use, then we are at risk. There is a brief history to each of these and you will be shocked at the reasoning behind why we still have them. The products we will look at are considered controversial and that's EXACTLY why we need to look at them. We have heard the mainstream argument for these things all our lives and now is the time for alternative answers. The things we will cover are genetically modified organisms (GMO's), fluoridated water, vaccinations, sugar, dairy, meat, smoking, alcohol, medications and what a person's attitude and emotion can do to one's health. You might think some of these are no brainers like alcohol and smoking, but trust me when I say every single thing mentioned here has something to offer on cancer causation and modern disease.

If you doubt or disbelieve any of these to be harmful or the cause of anything evil or insidious then I would say that's exactly the point. These products are designed to go under your radar so you do not perceive them as a threat, so keep an open mind and be prepared to re-educate yourself on some of the most important things we have taken for granted.

What are GMO's?

What if I told you that cancer doesn't have to be this bleak and morbid disease that everyone makes it out to be and that most diseases could be prevented? It sounds too good to be true but a famous quote by Linus Pauling, an American Biochemist and 2 times Nobel Peace prize winner, peace activist, educator and publisher of more than 1200 papers and 850 books on scientific issues said: "You can trace every sickness, every disease, and every ailment to a mineral deficiency." The human body is made up of 90 essential nutrients, 60 minerals, 16 vitamins, 12 amino acids and 2 essential fatty acids. These are the building blocks for making humans; these 90 essential nutrients are so essential that if they are not present in the mother during pregnancy then the baby is likely to suffer due to the lack of building material needed to construct a new child. So why are minerals so important to the human body? Minerals are vital because our bodies cannot make them on their own, we primarily get them from the plants we eat and the water we drink, the same plants that agricultural use chemical fertilizer, pesticide, herbicide and fungicide on. These chemicals kill the microorganisms living in the soil which are responsible for breaking down minerals which plants use to stay healthy, and what we ultimately eat. This is why it's a major problem and adds weight to the argument for why we are seeing an increase in all diseases and not just cancer.

So if you have strong opinions on any of these controversial subjects that we are about to look at then that's ok, but remember to have a valid opinion you must hear both sides of the argument, only then can you contribute to the debate.

That said in the interest of keeping an open mind I would like to share a quote with you from one of the greatest geniuses of all time and my personal favourite, Leonardo da Vinci. *Blinding ignorance does mislead us. O! Wretched mortals, open your eyes!*

The story you haven't heard

Who would have guessed that eating your fruit and vegetables would be bad for you when I researched this subject I quickly learned that not all foods are created equal and that 95% of the food in the supermarket was rubbish. For as long as I can remember my grandparents have always said "They" are messing around with the food, it's just not the same as the old days. I found this observation interesting because the diseases and disorders that are common today were rarities back in theirs, so maybe there was some truth to this. They would tell me that chicken used to be so dry and lean that you would have to baste it to keep it moist but now there is less protein and more fat in a standard bird and virtually no O-Mega 3 Fatty Acids, the flour used to be course and great but now it's bleached and as fine as talcum powder, eggs used to be fresh but now when you crack an egg it's as runny as water inside, and many other examples.

We have clearly done something different to bring on these enormous changes in the way we raise livestock and grow our fruit and vegetables. My grandparent's generation didn't have the internet, one of the greatest tools for research, information and communication in the 21st century, which is why these days we can get information on just about anything if we ask the right questions.

For those of you who do not know what genetically modified organisms are, it's where scientists take the gene from one organism and put it in another to utilise those specific characteristics. A good example of this is tomatoes, scientists took the gene from lemon basil and put it into a transgenic tomato to achieve better taste, 60% of people preferred the smell and taste of this tomato. Drought resistance is another example; this could be useful in most major crops such as corn, maize and soy grown in warmer climates or where rain is more unpredictable in countries like Australia which is known for long periods of drought.

Just to give you an idea of how far these biotech companies have taken genetic modification, they have also tried crossing spider genes with goats to produce silk, so when they milk the goat the silk produced could be used to make bulletproof vests. They have genetically modified salmon also called Frankenfish which if they ever got out would decimate the native population, they have even taken the glow in the dark gene in jellyfish and put it in mice as seen in this picture.

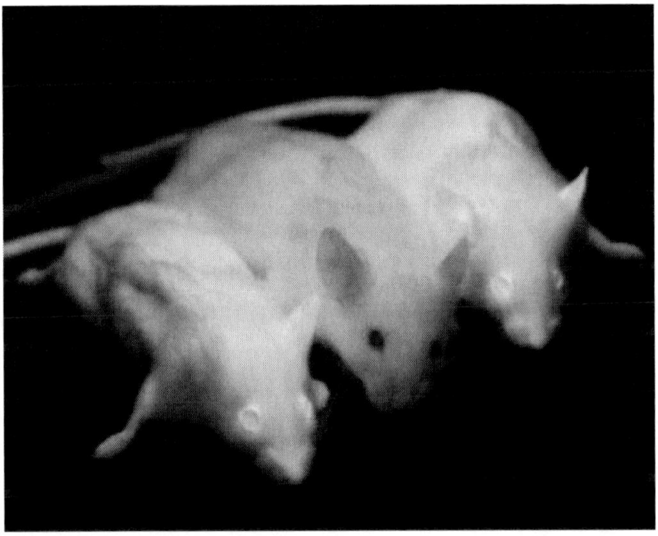

These biotech companies are trying to play God, the real question is why improve upon that which does not need improving? Everything in nature has a relationship with everything else and to disrupt that relationship is to invite chaos.

There are 2 major problems with GMO's particularly in plants; the first is that with any fruit, vegetable, grain, or tree is that they possess a natural pesticide called phytochemicals which are used to attack insects when they attack the plant. These chemical signals tell the plant to boost its natural insecticide to kill the attacker because plants cannot move like other organisms, the chemical is so strong that neighbouring plants get the message and start to boost their phytochemicals in response to the initial attack. If you have ever smelt freshly cut grass, then this is basically what you are smelling.

When scientists genetically modify a plant they modify it to produce significantly higher levels of phytochemicals, up to 3-4 times the norm which initially deters insects until they develop resistance in which case the process needs to be refined making the product more and more toxic. Consuming a crop which has been modified like this has a similar effect on people as it does the insect, it has toxic chemicals in the vegetable matter which are immune suppressants and cancer-causing which may also result in other diseases and disorders.

The second problem and by far the worst is that plants that have been genetically modified are also modified to withstand synthetic chemical pesticides, herbicides and fungicides sprayed externally on the plant. Due to the genetic modification, the plant absorbs these chemicals into the plant fibres without dying and in doing so these pesticides, herbicides and fungicides find their way into the fruit or vegetable that you are eating. Monsanto's specifically design their herbicide for the seeds they modify called roundup ready, but they have also genetically modified the plants to produce terminator seeds, meaning that when the plant matures and produces seeds of its own they won't grow, forcing farmers to go back to Monsanto's every year to buy new seeds for their crop.

When you buy fruit and vegetables at your supermarket, you may think it looks good, smells good and tastes good, so it must be good, right? Wrong! Catastrophically wrong! They say it's the punch you don't see that puts you down and it couldn't be truer with GMO's. At face value, it all sounds like butterflies and rainbows except the effect of these genetically modified organisms are a detriment to human health. The toxic chemical primarily used and responsible for cancer and many other disease and disorders in commercial agriculture is called is Glyphosate, which is so toxic and dangerous that senior research scientist Dr Stephanie Seneff from the Massachusetts Institute of Technology (MIT) said this.

"Glyphosate is possibly the most important factor in the development of multiple chronic diseases and conditions that have become prevalent in Westernized societies."

When GMO's first appeared there had been no independent short or long-term safety studies on GMO's or Glyphosate except for the initial study done for 6 weeks by Monsanto, which the FDA approved without any independent safety study. Since the introduction of GMO's into the marketplace studies have been linking Glyphosate to medical conditions such as cancer, massive liver and kidney damage, hormone problems, nutritional deficiencies, celiac disease, non-Hodgkin's lymphoma, birth defects, infertility and a heap more.

The lack of scientific research into this subject should be of serious concern to health authorities considering the scale of GMO foods in our diet today. But these government lapdogs seem to be too busy collecting paychecks from these companies to notice that GMO's could be the cause of anything insidious. Despite the overwhelming data warning of these hidden health dangers, these products remain at our local supermarket unregulated and undisclosed to the consumer about what kind of product they are buying.

We are told that there are no side effects from the consumption of these toxic products based on the lab results produced by Monsanto's, one of the largest genetically modified seed producers in the world. Government health departments run by former Monsanto's employees swear that there exists no evidence that genetically modified organisms are dangerous to human health based on a 90-day trial done on rats, and because there appeared to be no side effects in this 90-day trial, no human trials were warranted. The FDA's official statement on GMO's said that if there are no known side effects on GMO's, then they shall be treated like non-GMO. Does it make sense to you that a government department who is the authority on what is safe for people to eat would approve GMO's without ANY human testing? As many as 15 former Monsanto's employees have wormed their way into government health departments where at least 5 of them were appointed by the Obama administration.

Even Hillary Clinton is an advocator of GMO foods and would like to rebrand them so people are not afraid of them, but many reports say that she eats organic at home. Do what I say not what I do seems to be the message here and those that question Hilary Clinton's involvement with biotech companies like Monsanto's and Dow need only look at the generous donations she and others make to the Clinton Global Initiative (CGI), which is to gather world leaders on challenging global issues like how to feed 7.2 billion people.

In March 2010 Islam Siddiqui a former Monsanto's lobbyist was appointed to the position of the United States Trade Representative as the countries chief agricultural negotiator by the Obama administration. A position paper soon followed on behalf of the United States Department of Agriculture (USDA) and the Food and Drug Administration (FDA) claiming that it is false, misleading and deceptive to disclose whether food is genetically modified and strongly opposed to any kind of labelling for these kinds of products. Yes, you read that shit right! Government health departments do not want you to know what you are eating by not disclosing where or how your food was produced.

Most people like my parents refused to believe any of this, saying why doesn't someone do something about it? Oddly, that's the easy part, the people who are supposed to do something about it are in on the scam, so why change it if it's paying off? I am certainly no advocate of Hitler but he wasn't wrong when he said "tell a lie long enough and loud enough and anyone will believe it," because this has essentially become the motto of governments all over the world.

There appears to be a global plan with Monsanto's and that is to take over the world by being the sole proprietor of all things food. They are doing this by contaminating and destroying heirloom strains, infiltrating places in positions of power and they also have a thing for suing farmers for patent infringement when it is Monsanto's crops that have contaminated the farmers land. The farmer loses even if he wins because the purpose of this is to essentially bankrupt the farmer so they can no longer continue farming.

Monsanto's has sued 145 farmers and settled more than 700 cases outside of court within 16 years, it seems like an almost impossible feat but until recently they had never lost a case. It was only recently that Monsanto's was found guilty by a jury when their product Roundup Ready caused a school janitor in California cancer and was awarded 78 million dollars. In March 2019 a 70-year-old man called Edwin Hardeman also claimed that after 30 years of using Round-Up Ready that it caused is Non-Hodgkin's Lymphoma and are currently in the second stage of court proceedings for damages. Bayer one of the largest pharmaceutical companies in the world is currently looking at 11,000 similar cases in the US alone.

One of the earliest and most famous cases of Monsanto's contaminating a crop was with Canadian farmer Percy Schmeiser in 1997 when he suspected that Monsanto's had contaminated his canola crop by planting their GMO canola nearby. After spraying the crop and it not dying he realised that his crop had been contaminated by Monsanto's as it was now resistant to chemicals. He decided to save the seed separately from his other crops and replanted it the following year. Monsanto's came to Percy and said that he had to pay them a licence fee for using their patented product, but he argued that the seed was originally his and that they were at fault for contaminating his land, then on August 6 1998, Monsanto's sued Percy for patent infringement. After several years of going through the court system, a supreme court ruled in favour of Monsanto's because they held a valid patent and Percy knowingly replanted the GMO seed.

In 1999 Percy sued Monsanto's for millions for libel, trespass and contamination of his crops but this was dragged out to 2007 where he did not prosecute the lawsuit. In 2005 when Monsanto's had contaminated his fields he asked them to clean it up but Monsanto's refused unless he signed a confidentiality agreement to release them from litigation. The cost of the clean-up was $660 which Percy eventually sued Monsanto's in small claims court where Monsanto's finally paid. A drop in the bucket compared to the millions he should have won, but it just goes to show you that not even Percy Schmeiser who was the mayor of Bruno in Canada from 1966-1983 stood a chance against this company and since then they have been a nightmare to every farmer that has ever crossed paths with them.

Globally more than 100 million acres of transgenic crops will be used to perpetuate the global genetic pollution problem which cannot be contained. Only 30 years ago more than 800 million people were growing their food and as more farmers are forced off their land by corporations like Monsanto's this will only get worse. Companies like Monsanto's are buying up farmers land like you won't believe and are contributing to starvation by killing diversity and they are doing it just to grow this toxic shit we now call the Green Revolution.

Monsanto's Real Identity

It all started with the Vietnam war between 1961 and 1971 with the militaries chemical weapon program, the star of this program was a chemical weapon called Agent Orange, called that because of the bright orange stripes displayed on the canisters that contained it. The US military commissioned Monsanto's, Dow and a few other major chemical companies to develop a chemical weapon comprised of highly toxic herbicides. Agent Orange was a combination of 2 highly concentrated herbicides 2,4-D and 2,4,5-T that if used separately would only be toxic for a couple of days, however, combined they had a toxic by-product called dioxin, Its chemical name is 2,3,7,8-tetrachloro-dibenzo-para-dioxin, or TCDD, which included PCBs that today we know are cancer-causing, yet dioxin was the most toxic out of 419 similar toxic compounds. The US Air Force began test spraying on August 10, 1961, which gave the green light for Operation Ranch Hand, the operations mission was to destroy the enemy's food supply using Agent Orange and to drive or starve the Vietnamese out of Southern Vietnam.

Operation Ranch Hand went from 1962 to 1971 whereas much as 24% of southern Vietnam was exposed to this toxic chemical in concentrations as much as 50 times higher than what was needed for the desired effect. During the time of this spraying, a study found that 3,181 villagers were sprayed, 5 million acres of mangroves were destroyed and 500,000 acres of crops were destroyed as well as the borders of Laos and Cambodia.

As much as 43 million litres of Agent Orange were dumped during Operation Ranch Hand and the effects of this chemical weapon are still being felt in Vietnam today. The half-life of its toxicity in humans is between 11-15 years but can be as high as 20 years on surfaces such as plants and soil and if leached into the deep sediment of rivers it can be as long as 100 years.

Any claims that the military, Monsanto's, Dow and the other chemical companies involved did not know about the side effects of this chemical weapon is absolute bullshit, concentrations of 50 times anything that is already poisonous is going to kill you. It sounds to me like the military were desperate to win a losing war and the need for a game changer gave precedence over the sanctity of human life whether it be casualties of war such as villagers not directly caught up in the fight, or the military's personnel, not too mention the environmental impact that continues today. They mustn't have thought too long about potential consequences because it all happened pretty quickly and to some degree, this was confirmed by Dr James Clary the designer for the herbicide spray tank at the chemical weapons branch of Elgin Air Force Base when he told Senator Daschle in 1988 the following:

"When we (military scientists) initiated the herbicide program in the 1960s, we were aware of the potential for damage due to dioxin contamination in the herbicide. We were even aware that the 'military' formulation had a higher dioxin concentration than the 'civilian' version due to the lower cost and speed of manufacture.

However, because the material was to be used on the 'enemy,' none of us were overly concerned. We never considered a scenario in which our own personnel would become contaminated with the herbicide."~ Quoted by Admiral Elmo R. Zumwalt, 1990.

The casualties of this weapon's use are estimated between 2.1 and 4.5 million Vietnamese civilians; the U.S Veterans Administration presumes as many as 2.8 million Americans were exposed and the Vietnamese Red Cross estimates 3 million Vietnamese exposed 150,000 of which are the results of birth defects from exposure to Agent Orange.

These are the kind of birth defects the Vietnamese people have had live with to this day. (See Page 123)

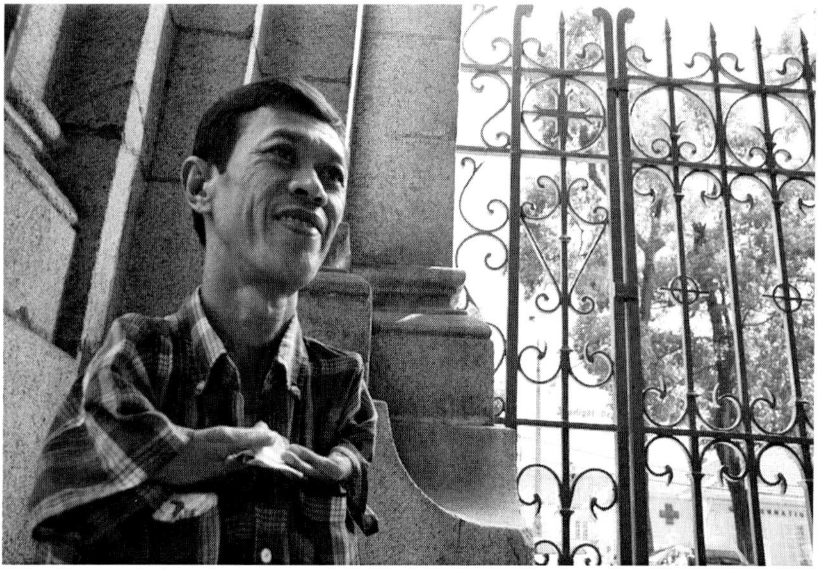

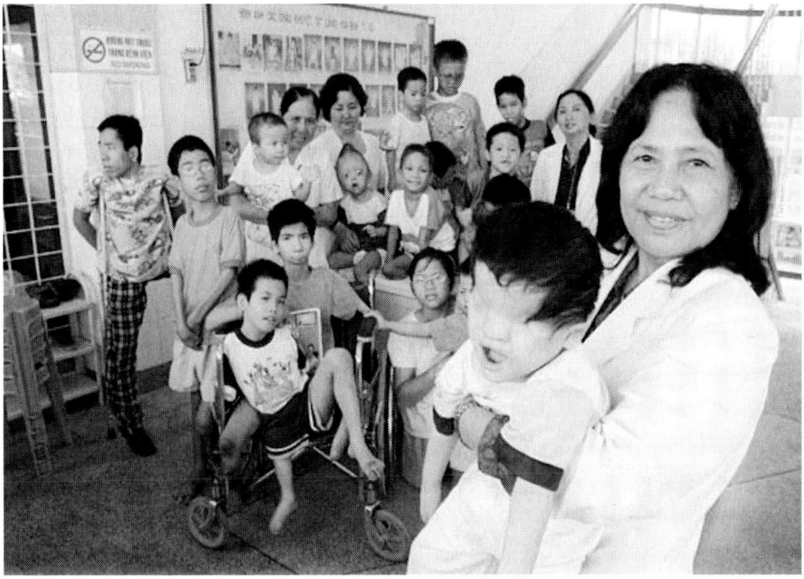

The New & Improved Monsanto's

Because of Monsanto's involvement with the US Military and their creation of chemical weapons, Monsanto's had attracted a lot of negative publicity. That was until the arrival of Mitt Romney, an American businessman and politician who ran Bain Capital, an alternative finance group. Monsanto's became Bain Capitals biggest client, this multi-million dollar relationship lasted between 1977 and 1985 and benefited both organizations enormously. Due to the negative image Monsanto's created, it was Mitt Romney who suggested a shift towards biotechnology and the development of chemical herbicides used for commercial agricultural purposes. Dr Earl Beaver Monsanto's waste director during the 70s and 80s said that Romney was the major driving proponent in the shift to the biotechnical and bioengineering industry. Romney has received from agribusinesses like Monsanto's more than $4,075,531 in campaign contributions, whereas Barack Obama had only taken

$1,377,503, even though both clearly have a love GMO's. It remains as clear as day that as long as politicians like these keep getting donations of this magnitude from corrupt corporations, it's unlikely that things will change as man seldom chooses the higher path over financial gain.

Due to Romney's influence, Monsanto's went from the development of chemicals weapons used in warfare to genetically modifying organisms and putting food on your table by using their herbicides and pesticides both of which contain Glyphosate. In case you haven't caught on yet "Glyphosate is the new and improved agent orange" just look at the similarities between the following diseases and disorders that are associated with Agent Orange and what scientists are saying GMO's and Glyphosate cause.

Disease	Agent Orange	GMO + Glyphosate
ADHD		✓
Allergies		✓
ALS		✓
Alzheimer's disease		✓
Autism		✓
Birth Defects	✓	✓
Brain Cancer	✓	✓
Breast Cancer	✓	✓
Cancers (Other)	✓	✓
Cardiovascular Disease		✓
Chloracne	✓	✓
Chron's Disease		✓
Depression		✓
Hodgkin 's disease	✓	✓
IBS		✓
Infertility	✓	✓
Multiple Myeloma	✓	
Multiple Sclerosis		✓
Non-Hodgkin's Lymphoma	✓	✓
Nutritional Deficiencies	✓	✓

Obesity		✓
Parkinson's	✓	✓
Porphyria	✓	
Prostate Cancer	✓	✓
Respiratory Cancers	✓	✓
Respiratory Issues	✓	✓
Reproductive Problems	✓	✓
Soft tissue Carcinoma	✓	

The Real Research

In 2009 a French court found Monsanto's guilty of lie labelling its herbicide as biodegradable, environmentally friendly and that there were no traces left in the soil. An enormous amount of evidence now points at Monsanto and their use of glyphosate, even the Environmental Protection Agency (EPA) in the 1980s officially said that glyphosate should be a class C carcinogen but they were pressured by Monsanto's to retract this statement and change their assessment which is now the complete opposite to what they originally said. The World Health Organization (WHO) has also said that there is serious potential for cancer to develop specifically Non-Hodgkin's lymphoma but it seems that all Monsanto's has to do to keep their products on the shelf is simply disagree with the science and say there are no risks.

In November 2012 the Journal of Food and Chemical Toxicology published a paper called the Long-Term Toxicity of Roundup Herbicide and a Roundup-Tolerant genetically modified maize by researcher and molecular biologist professor Gilles-Eric Seralini and his research team at the France Caen University. The paper showed the long-term toxicity from Monsanto's GMO Maize and the use of the NK603 glyphosate-based herbicide roundup and received global attention. The journal retracted the paper after being published claiming that Gilles-Eric Seralini and his team didn't use the correct strain of rats to conduct their research, but Seralini argued that it was irrelevant because he used the same strain and number of test rats that Monsanto's did to push their approval through, apples for apples so to speak. It was only after 9 months did the rats showed the long-term side effects of GMO's and glyphosate which resulted in tumours and other serious life-threatening conditions.

He further added that Monsanto's tests only went for 90 days which wasn't long enough to determine anything, Seralini's test was done over 2 years and concluded that Monsanto's products should have never hit the shelves.

Another study on the effects of GMO's was called *"A Comparison of the Effects of Three GM Corn Varieties on Mammalian Health"*. It took 3 of Monsanto's GM corn varieties and studied the long-term effects of consuming it alongside trace amounts of Monsanto's chemical roundup fertilizer. Believe it or not, the study was deemed the most thorough research ever published into the health effects of GM food crops and the herbicide Roundup on rats. The outcome of their findings was unbelievable, resulting in widespread organ damage, tumours so large that they even had trouble breathing, and a premature death rate of 50% in males and 70% in females. The rats had also developed mammary tumours, severe liver & kidney damage in as early as 4 months, and the rats that drank trace amounts of roundup the same amount legally allowed into the water supply showed an increase in tumour size of 200% to 300%.

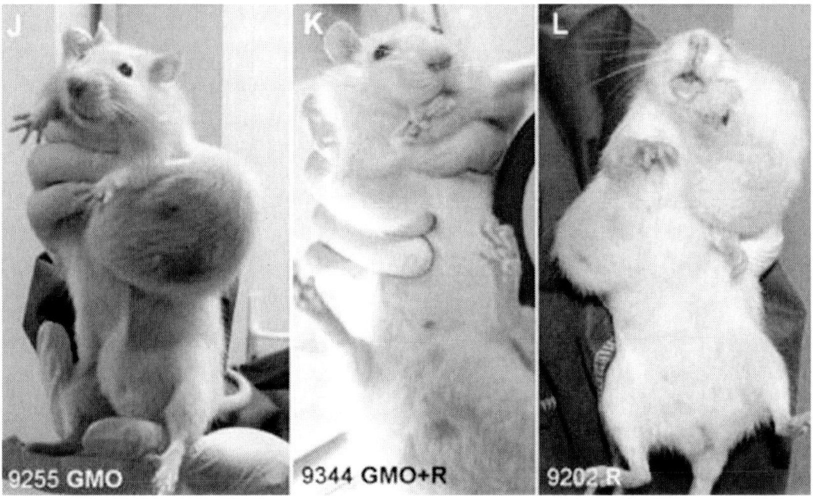

When I contacted Seralini and his team for research on this book I absolutely had to get these images, words just seem inadequate to describe that every time you are eating fruit and vegetables from your supermarket you are consuming the same chemicals that led to these rats condition.

These rats were fed on Monsanto's NK603 GM variety of corn, the same variety of corn that was widely fed to livestock and used in corn-based breakfast cereals, corn tortillas and corn snack chips. If you would like to see more of Professor Seralini's research and discover more about GMO's then you can go to www.gmoseralini.org.

Below are two quotes from Dr Michael Antoniou, a molecular biologist at King's College London about his involvement with the study.

"This research shows an extraordinary number of tumours developing earlier and more aggressively – particularly in female animals.

I am shocked by the extreme negative health impacts!

"We can expect that the consumption of GM maize and the herbicide Roundup, impacts seriously on human health".

Many other studies are showing the long-term side effects of consuming GMO's and Glyphosate, a research team in Canada conducted a study and published it in the Journal of Reproductive Toxicology in 2011. Their findings showed the presence of Monsanto's BT Toxin (a pesticide) in maternal, fetal and non-pregnant women's blood. The study tested 30 pregnant and non-pregnant woman and found the fetus is extremely susceptible to the effects of xenobiotics. Xenobiotics are chemical's produced by an organism that is not natural like those found in GM foods and because of the unknown effects on the ecology of the body and fetus they concluded more research needed to be done to deem them safe.

Another tactic used by large companies to persuade the masses that the science supports their arguments is the tactic of "Ghost Writing" and Monsanto's are experts at it. This works when Monsanto's gets one of their scientists to write a study word for word on how GMO's and Glyphosate is safe, then they approach an institution like a university department that needs funding and says "we will give you $100,000 if you publish this study word for word". This is exactly why the information in the scientific community can be so ambiguous and make issues like GMO's and Glyphosate safety seem complex when in reality they're not.

GMO's are also devastating to our environment which indirectly affects our health. The BT corn strain is so toxic that the pollen kills monarch butterflies, bees, but also any insect that has a larval form or alkaline gut.

It is estimated that if all pollinating insects were to die humans would only live for 3 years before global extinction, we are that dependant on them, yet GMO's remain. If GMOs were discussed as much as terrorism or whos screwing who on reality TV then perhaps it would be getting the attention it deserves, but it would seem that just getting the public to acknowledge it's a problem is the biggest obstacle so far.

Removing GMO's from your diet

To remove GMO's from your diet there are a couple of solutions. The most cost-effective one in the long term is to grow your own organic heirloom strain vegetables. This can be done by jumping online and buying the seeds of plants you commonly eat, you will want a wide variety of plants as they grow in different seasons and you can use the supermarket to fill the gaps with organic fruit and vegetables that are out of that season. Furthermore, always use organic soils and fertilisers and always research what it contains before using it on the plants you plan to eat. Most young people think of gardening as a pastime for old people, but it is one of the most rewarding activities you can do. You cannot beat a homegrown tomato and the taste and smell is something a store-bought tomato cannot capture.

Pest control is another issue when growing your own but this can be easily managed by mixing some strong chilies and garlic in water with a bit of cooking oil, filtering it out and spraying it on the leaves, this should have insects buzzing for the hills. You can also plant plants that invite predatory insects like ladybugs to control things like aphids which reproduce insanely fast. It's important that chemical-free means exactly that, so no chemical fertilizers for your lawn either. If your children or pets play on the lawn where chemical fertilizers and sprays have been used it could be potentially harmful.

The other option is, if growing your own seems too laborious for you or you have limited space then I suggest potting vegetables or finding your local market or greengrocer and look for GMO-free labelling if you can find it, you can always buy organic if you cannot grow your own, but the variety of foods will be limited.

The 100% shop method raises the issues of cost, and organic can get costly which should tell you how insane this all is because organic is how food is supposed to be, not genetically modified, and now you have to pay more for healthier food. Unfortunately, GMO's will find their way into your diet somehow, they are in so many products now that it's impossible to stop it without going to the source and by taking these measures you are making a huge difference to the biochemistry of your body and can feel a real sense of relief knowing you're making a stand for toxic-free food.

The solution to this problem is within the people's power and by learning what is in your food you can take back what was forced upon you without our consent and not burden future generations with a lifetime of disease and disorders due to our complacency and unwillingness for change. If you find yourself still questioning GMO's then perhaps you would take more from the documentary called "GMO seeds of Death" produced by Gary Null, this will shed some more insight into the GMO issue and solidify what you have learned here. Also, there are many authors out there on this subject, one that may be of particular interest is Carey Gilliam called "White Wash – the story of a weed killer, cancer and the corruption of science". If you are looking for more scientific research on GMO's and Glyphosate then Dr Stephanie Seneff's website would be a great place to start, at www.people.csail.mit.edu/seneff.

Final Caution: If you are buying seeds online to start your own Green Revolution, do not get them from eBay or Amazon as most of them come from China, I have seen many GMO seeds titled heirloom misleadingly. Instead, support your local seed producer and buy locally or nationally.

CHAPTER 9: FLUORIDE! MEDICATING THE MASSES!

There is a strong belief in the remaining few countries around the world that continue to fluoridate their water supply that it is essential for preventing tooth decay and sadly that is what we are expected to believe. Approximately 5% of the world's population drinks fluoridated water which translates to roughly 370,000,000 people in approximately 25 countries such as Australia (80%), Brunei (95%); Chile (70%), Guyana (62%), Hong Kong (100%), the Irish Republic (73%), Israel (70%), Malaysia (75%), New Zealand (62%), Singapore (100%) and the United States (64%) where their consumption is above 50%. Despite the official explanation, there is a growing body of evidence that fluoride is toxic to human health and this evidence has been amounting every single year. Governments around the world who continue this pointless and dangerous practice have consistently argued that insufficient evidence exists to support claims of human health dangers to fluoridating the water supply. On the other hand independent labs, researchers, dentists and many others have consistently supplied evidence to support their claims, evidence which is ignored by the regulatory authorities and so the debate continues. A major reason why health authorities ignore the evidence on issues like fluoride is that of accountability. If governments were held accountable after it was proven that they knew it was damaging to human health it would turn their people against them and they would not be able to control the outrage. It would also violate their number one policy for controlling the masses, which is to lie and deny everything as most governments do.

If you are new to the fluoride debate you will need to understand the difference between calcium fluoride (CaF2) and sodium fluoride (NaF), a distinction rarely made by authorities or the corporations selling this crap in the name of water treatment. The difference between these two compounds has been heavily skewed by the corporations by deceiving the public into thinking they are both the same especially ALCOA, who is the Aluminium Company of America. There are a few compounds of fluoride, calcium fluoride is a mineral found naturally in soil and rock which is relatively harmless to people, but sodium fluoride is a synthetic manmade waste product from the aluminium, steel, fertilizer and even the nuclear industry.

According to Mike Adams also known as the health ranger who is an activist turned scientist and promoter of holistic and alternative medicine, sodium fluoride is an umbrella term for as many as 100 toxic chemicals some of which are known to cause cancer and a whole range of other health problems. Some of these chemicals and heavy metals are arsenic, aluminium, cadmium, fluorosilicic acid, lead, mercury and even some radioactive materials. Only a small amount of sodium fluoride is needed to kill you and its toxicity pound for pound rivals that of rat poison, which is funny because its an ingredient in rat poison. Fluorine compounds such as hydrofluoric acid and other toxic chemicals are used to refine high octane gas, make plastics, semiconductors, screen's and even toothpaste all of which find their way into the water you drink and wash in every day. Sodium fluoride is also an ingredient in pesticides, insecticides and fungicides, all of which is used on the foods we buy at the supermarket and use in our gardens.

After learning just some of the things that fluoride is in, you can already surmise what this could be doing to your health, and what were the benefits again? Preventing tooth decay? That sounds lovely, except its all bullshit! I'm sure you would agree that you would rather have a cavity in your tooth than a cocktail of dangerous poisons in your drinking water which you use every day. To put what happened into context you will need to hear how fluoride got into your water in the first place and for that we will need to go back to ALCOA.

The History of Fluoride

The history of Fluoride is a mile long so I will try to wrap up all the important points so that you get the picture of where this lie came from. According to author Christopher Bryson who wrote the book called "The Fluoride Deception", the first suggestion that fluoride could be good for your teeth was in a letter from Francis Freire who was the director of the Aluminium Laboratory for the Aluminium Company of America (ALCOA). The letter was addressed to Gerald J Cox at the Melon Institute in Pitts burg who raised concerns about fluorides toxicity to the environment and people of the community especially ALCOA's workers. ALCOA claimed that there appeared to be some dental benefits to using fluoride and so Gerald J Cox and the Melon Institute started to look into it, they magically concluded that there were dental benefits and began promoting its use with very little if any actual evidence to support their claims.

The Melon Institute also has a history of defending the use of asbestos, so that might give you some insight as to why I would be sceptical about their claims.

The Melon Institute and Cox were so sure that it did what they claimed without affecting people's health that in 1939 Cox publicly stated the following.

The present trend towards complete removal of fluoride from water and food may need some reversal.

By 1957 the trend of fluoridating everything started to gain momentum and a distinguished toxicologist by the name of Harold Hodge claimed that fluoride at 1 part per million is safe and possess no risk to human health and that it should be added to the drinking water without delay. The very same Harold Hodge was also a co-founder of the human radiation experiment where he oversaw a team of scientists inject plutonium and uranium into hospital patients. Harold Hodge was also the chief toxicologist in the Manhattan Project which was the project for the development of the nuclear bomb. Hodges job was to determine the toxicity of the chemicals used in the production of nuclear weapons and guess what chemical they need shitloads of? Fluoride...

ALCOA was producing enormous amounts of waste (Sodium Fluoride) that they were burying it in toxic landfills and poisoning the environment, they were desperate to find a solution as toxic landfill is extremely expensive to dispose of due to its environmental impact. Perhaps at the time, they were thinking along the lines of John Adams who is one of America's founding fathers who famously said that "every problem is an opportunity in disguise".

So ALCOA hired Dr Henry Trendley Dean who was the first director of the United States National Institute of Dental

Research to go to more than 300 cities to see if he could find a link between tooth decay and fluoride, not one single city showed any correlations. There were however approximately 28 out of these 300 cities that showed less tooth decay but a higher rate of fluorosis, so ALCOA interpreted that to mean that fluoride must work, so after pondering on this so-called revelation in their smoke-filled room, they were thinking how the hell do we sell this bullshit to the masses? Until they had an ah-ha moment and realized that they don't, so they hired a guy called Edward Bernays who wrote the bestselling book "Propaganda", which was all about how to brainwash the masses without them knowing. Edward Bernay's just happens to be the nephew of Sigmund Freud the father of psychology, so its no fucking wonder people think fluoride is good for them. I first heard this from another researcher and advocate of natural and alternative medicine called Ty Bollinger who wrote the book "Cancer, step outside the box", who is a lot more conservative in his writing than I am, so if you prefer something less blunt and in your face, he would be a good choice.

The history of fluoride reads like a horror story and if I hadn't researched it myself I would have never believed it! According to senior scientist, Dr Edward Groth between 1957 and 1968 fluoride was responsible for more damage to industry than all 20 nationally monitored air pollutants combined. It is said that fluoride was even used by Hitler because of its primary effect to dumb people down and take away their will to resist, though many people still debate whether it was used during WWII. It always made me wonder if countries like Australia which are so massively overregulated and taxed, is fluoridated to stop people from protesting the unjust oppression they are under. Especially when you can get fined more than $200 for littering simply by emptying a bottle of water on to the ground which is exactly what happened to Melbourne truckie Michael Hagen in 2012. Is this the reason why we still fluoridate our water supply, to ensure our compliance by drugging us and sapping our will to resist such ridiculous laws? It's an interesting and intriguing thought and if the current COVID 19 situation hasn't taught people that the political class will say and do anything no matter how illogical it seems then frankly I don't know what anyone could say to make them smell the roses! I know one thing for sure, if half of what is written here was common knowledge then there is no way the general population would sit back and put up with their lies. We would see a version of the yellow vest movement here in Australia which dare I say needs to happen if real change is to occur. Just think about the ramifications if it was known all along that fluoride is a dangerous poison and was knowingly put into the water supply. There would be riots, protests, lawsuits, class actions, compensation claims you name it, not to mention a complete loss of faith in government, not like there's any left.

Perhaps the reason the few remaining countries still fluoridate their water has something to do with Cargill, which is not only the largest producer of hydrofluorosilicic acid but is the largest privately owned corporation in the world with a revenue of more than 134 billion dollars. Governments buy this shit as a product, and because places like China stopped fluoridating their water supply, now we buy it off them because it's cheaper poison than buying it domestically.

Fluorides history is enormous and there are many books out there warning people about its toxicity, I am always learning something new about this subject and the more I learn the more I realise how integrated this chemical is in the remaining countries that still use it. We are supposed to believe that fluoride is in the water to prevent tooth cavities and poses no human health risks, but if that's the case then why do some toothpaste's that contain fluoride have a warning that says do not swallow and if ingested to contact your local poison control centre. Think about it, if fluoride is so harmless then what's the difference between fluoride in your water and fluoride in your toothpaste? Most people don't think this is a serious issue, but like most things, people don't hear enough about it to know why they should worry.

There is no way on earth the Australian government doesn't know exactly what this chemical does because they have the exact same information as the countries that stopped using it. For some reason beyond all explanation Australia is in the stone age on issues like these because while we are still using this chemical the majority of Europe has banned fluoride and even GMO's because they know that if something has the potential to cause harm whether it is known 100% or not you don't give it to people and hope for the best.

We are now seeing the effects of a toxic environment in our children and young adults, getting diseases and disorders that are normally quite rare or not seen until much later in life which is a typical sign of bioaccumulation or high-level exposure. Continuous gradual exposure leads to increased risk especially for children and teenagers in their developing years and that's because their hormones have not balanced out which is where a lot of the damage occurs.

For the last 10 years, I have used fluoride-free toothpaste or some other alternative and in that time I have only had 1 small tooth cavity. Also, I distil my water and if you want to see exactly what comes out of your tap water at home then brace yourself because you are about to have an illuminating experience.

Below is what came out of 4 litres of standard tap water.

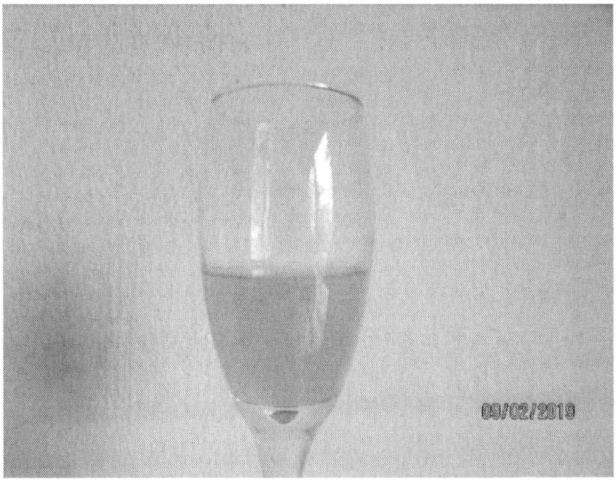

After 24 hours of letting the water stand this is the accumulation on the bottom. It had a rotten pipe smell and was absolutely vile!

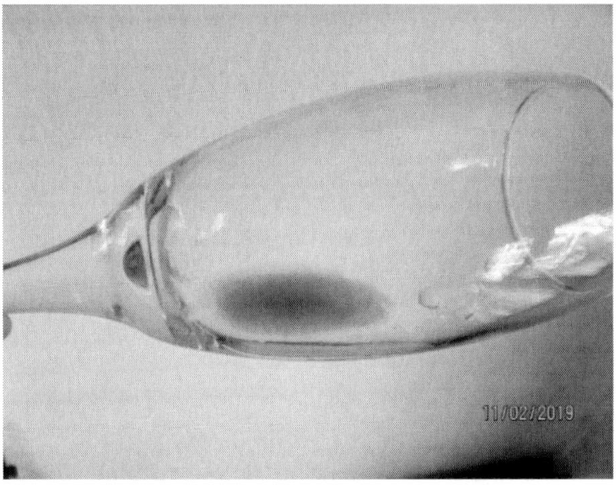

I always knew the drinking water was bad and I try to drink filtered water whenever I can, but the severity of this was confirmed in 2018 when I was a residential property manager and a tenant complained that their tap water was contaminated after distilling it. I knew exactly what was in the water and for the first time in a long time, it was reassuring to see someone just as concerned as me. I had Westernport water check the mains of the property for contamination and also check the house to see if it was inside. After showing me a glass of water distilled from 4 litres it was no better than mine from home, so I sent the images to Westernport water so they could test the water supply. After a week I was told directly by them that the level of contaminants is within the acceptable tolerance of their safety protocols for standard tap water, then they tried to sell me some bullshit on how if I distil my water I would be losing minerals and fluoride for my teeth. These people actually think that these are selling points, to this day I am convinced that if you have the IQ of a dishcloth and the attention span of a moth, then you will get a job in Government and places like this. This is why getting any meaningful answers anywhere today is practically impossible, everyone has been indoctrinated. Whatever minerals may have been present would have been offset by the numerous contaminants in the water, you wouldn't shot a cocktail of deadly poisons and say to yourself, if I eat an apple for its minerals I'll be ok! For 2 years I stopped using toothpaste altogether and used bicarb soda and not one filling or cavity in that time, so clearly my own experience has taught me that if you test the things you are told then sometimes the results will surprise you. Our diet, especially the westernized diet, has always been the source of tooth decay and if you compare that too indigenous cultures who have a varied diet away from processed foods and grains, then they have better dental hygiene than most western societies today. In Australia, the aboriginal people had some of the best teeth in all native tribes around the world which was due to a high diet of seafood's and traditionally charcoal and various antibacterial plants like Aloe Vera has been used to clean teeth way before toothbrushes and toothpaste came into the picture.

According to the World Health Organization between 1970 and 2010 the countries that stopped fluoridating their water supply experienced the same decline in child dental decay as the countries that continued. There should have been a greater decline in the countries that stopped fluoridate their water but this was not observed at all, demonstrating the true effectiveness of fluoride on tooth decay. Yet the World Health Organization still supports its use!

As I mentioned earlier the fluoride that ends up in our drinking water is a waste product of the aluminium, steel and fertilizer industry, this is done by quarrying huge amounts of rock and putting it into large vats where it is broken down using chemicals like sulfuric acid to extract the phosphates which are then used for chemical fertiliser. Deceptions like this one for corporations to profit are going on all the time, recently in Australia, we had the plastic bag ban where instead of getting bags for free, they made us buy reusable bags which even included plastic bags of slightly better quality. In other words, the supermarkets wanted us to pay for bags all along and so they sold us a whole bunch of bullshit about how they care about the environment to then justify the change only to bring plastic bags back except now we pay for them.

I have always said to never underestimate how gullible and naive the public can be when they are told the cause is for the greater good, people believe that the supermarkets care about the environment which is why this change was suggested in the first place, but it was just a tactic for supermarkets to reduce their costs.

Based on my research and the research of others far more established in this controversial issue the facts appear to be largely against fluoride, then again you don't have to believe me or anyone else just look at the countries that stopped adding it to their water supply. I mean if the stuff is so great why did they stop? Are we in Australia so arrogant to think that our studies on fluoride toxicity are the only ones that matter? The National Cancer Institute says on their website under the section "does fluoridated water cause cancer", that in 1990 a study by the National Toxicology Program which is part of the National Institute of Environmental Health Sciences, showed that male rats given high amounts of fluoride for 2 years increased the number of osteosarcomas (bone tumours). Yet they claim that studies done on humans showed no associations between fluoridated water and cancer in humans.

However, Eric Lander, director of the Whitehead Institute Centre for Genomic Research in Cambridge, Massachusetts said: "About 99% of genes in humans have their counterparts in the mouse" he further added that mice and humans share 30,000 genes of which 300 are unique to each species, we even share the gene for a tail, but it is turned off in humans. So how can humans and mice share 99% of their genes and yet fluoride on rats cause osteosarcomas, but not in mice and humans? This makes no sense at all!

My argument here was validated in a way by Dr Dean Burk who discovered that biotin is essential for cellular respiration, which is proper cell growth and the body's ability to carry out its normal metabolic functions.

Biotin is seriously impeded by the presence of fluoride and other toxins. Dr Burk was the head chief chemist at the National Cancer Institute and part of the National Institute of Health under the U.S. Department of Health and Human Services. Dr Burk had won the Hilderbrand Prize in 1952 for his work on photosynthesis and the Gerhard Domgak prize in 1965 for the development of procedures for distinguishing the difference between a normal cell and one damaged by cancer. So basically, Dr Burk knew his shit! He went on to say the following about the subject of enzyme disassociation and fluoride:

> *"In point of fact, fluoride causes more human cancer deaths than any other chemical. When you have power you don't have to tell the truth. That's a rule that's been working in this world for generations. And there are a great many people who don't tell the truth when they are in power in administrative positions. Fluoride amounts to public murder on a grand scale. It is some of the most conclusive scientific and biological evidence that I have come across in my 50 years in the field of cancer research."*

The Side Effects

There are many studies out there showing the negative health effects of fluoride and its impact on human health, particularly on the brain including an increased chance of autism, dementia and learning difficulties in children. In a published study called the *"Effect of Fluoridated water on intelligence in 10-12-year-old school children"* by Dr A Aravind at the Department of Public Health Dentistry, Al Azhar Dental College, Thodupuzha, Kerala in India, concluded that children's IQ level was seriously impacted by the level of fluoride found in drinking water and that it also can be toxic to many organ systems. In fact, to the best of my knowledge there are as many as 53 studies to date that show a connection between fluoride and reduced IQ in children, so why isn't this talked about more in the mainstream media?

As Mike Adams mentions that fluoride is an umbrella term for as many as 100 toxic chemicals, then there is no telling what chemical or heavy metal could be contributing to your current condition. We learned earlier that oxybenzone in sunscreen is in our tap water so God only knows what else could be coming through. Other side effects may include many cancer types, fluorosis which is often misdiagnosed as arthritis as the symptoms are very similar, diabetes, gastrointestinal problems, kidney disease, cardiovascular disease, endocrine disruptions, fertility problems, thyroid problems, hypersensitivity, pineal gland calcification and many more.

We know that many scientists and doctors acknowledge the dangers of fluoride and are making a stand for its removal.

The world's leading authority and number one critic for its use in our water is Dr Paul Connett. He was a founder of the fluoride action network and is where I would recommend starting if you want to get educated on this subject as it is quite involved. In one interview Dr Paul Connett mentioned that when he spoke with the ministry of health in New Zealand that he told them to write a scientific critic proving that the arguments made in his book "The Case Against Fluoride" which were based on scientific studies demonstrating fluorides harmful effects on people were wrong.

To date, they have never replied to this request! Dr Paul Connett has continued to be a leading figure in the fluoride debate worldwide and has done more than 2500 presentations on this dangerous chemical.

Fluoride is not just used in water it is found in many products such as medications, particularly those used for depression like Paxil and Prozac. However, there have been many medications that were removed where fluoride and fluoride compounds were responsible for their harmful side effects due to the potentially lethal doses. In 2000, Cisapride (Propulsid) a medication used for gastrointestinal issues was withdrawn because it caused severe cardiac side effects, Mibefradil (Posicor) a medication used for hypertension and chronic angina pectoris was withdrawn in 1998 when it was shown that patients with congestive heart failure had a higher mortality rate, or how about Tolrestat an anti-diabetic drug which was withdrawn in 1997 after it caused severe liver damage and deaths and I could go on and on, all medications with fluoride at their core.

Fluoride can also cross the placenta and affect the tissues of a developing fetus, the full effects of this are currently unknown but it is not unreasonable to say that they are not good based on what we already know. It has also been shown that babies that are breastfed are exposed to low concentrations of fluoride at roughly 0.004ppm, but a child who is bottle-fed is getting a fluoride dose 250 times through bottled formula where normal tap water is being used. Fluoride accumulates in the pineal gland which sits in between the 2 hemispheres of your brain, it is light sensitive and produces melatonin a wonder chemical that combats ageing, disease, cancer and all sorts of other problems in the body.

It only functions at night during deep sleep and fluoride directly interferes with its ability to function properly.

So does fluoride prevent cavities? Even if it did with some of the side effects mentioned here would you really want it? I would like to think that I have made a convincing argument to at least have you question whether your tap water is safe. The only way we are going to get rid of it is for everyone to come together on this problem and demands its removal. Fluoride is nothing more than mass medication and is the only drug in the world where the dose isn't controlled. People don't realize that it is an attack on your freedom to choose what you want to put into your body whether you think it is harmful or not.

The Solution

Do not be disheartened by this grim outlook because there are options available. If you go online you can pick up a distiller or a reverse osmosis filter for your home for under $200 and its a sound investment. I have a distiller, I add a little bit of pink Himalayan salt to the water after it has been filtered to add minerals back in and from my very first drink the taste and texture of the water were completely different. The best way to describe the difference is that of coarse water with smooth water, of course being both liquids I realize how this sounds but I promise you will notice a difference. If you're a big tea or coffee drinker then you will also want to get a new kettle that is completely glass or metal, not plastic. Just as a distiller boils water and collects the vapour your kettle also boils water and this is what all of the crap in your tap cooked on to the bottom looks like.

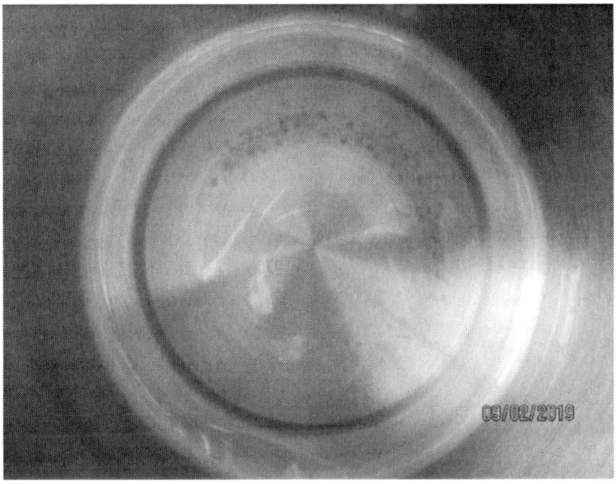

For the recovering cancer patient, this is an absolute must, mainly because you will want to keep fluids high especially if you have already had treatment. Up to 60% of the body is water, so if you have had chemo the toxins in your body will be high, so to reduce the impact you will need to dilute those toxins by staying hydrated with water you know is clean and mineral-rich.

For additional research into this issue, I would recommend the documentary "The Great Culling: Our water" by Paul Wittenberger which you can YouTube, it goes into more detail and explains how fluoridating the water supply may actually be part of a depopulation agenda to an out of control population crisis and is definitely worth a watch.

You can also get Dr Paul Connett's book "The Case Against Fluoride" or YouTube many of his videos. Finally, there is the Fluoride Action Network at www.fluoridealert.org where you can read articles, facts, recent news and even vote on how you feel about this chemical.

CHAPTER 10: VACCINATION! A KILLER COCKTAIL!

This is considered to be highly controversial and regardless of whether you agree or not I set out to raise awareness on cancer and modern disease, so I don't care if I tread on any toes here. All I want is to tell you how it is, the way it should have been told to you in the beginning, so let me simplify what's going on. When it comes time for you or your children to get their flu shots whether it's for hepatitis, measles, mumps, rubella, rotavirus, influenza A & B, swine flu, bird flu or whatever else you believe vaccines will fix, the keyword here is "Belief". The facts are that vaccines do not work in the way you are told and can be very dangerous especially to young children, pregnant women and the elderly. This has everything to do with the ingredients used in vaccines and how the immune system responds to them. Like the other subjects covered so far we have been sold a lie and the masses have not only bought it hook line and sinker, but they have swallowed the whole rod, reel and all.

The evidence on vaccine ingredients like thimerosal which is a mercury compound is something we are told is safe and is one of the greatest lies you are told when your doctor says a vaccine will cause you or your child no harm. Mercury is a known human carcinogen and extremely cellular toxic so why would a compound of mercury be any safer? It is primarily used in vaccines to prevent the growth of dangerous microbes, but what I always wondered was how does the virus or disease that you are trying to be immune to which is also a dangerous microbe survive in the presence of this compound?

This was a question I felt was inadequately explained by pro-vax and anti-vax people alike, but after a bit of research, I got my answer.

There are 2 types of vaccines that are used, one is replicating vaccines where the diseases are alive, and the other is non-replicating vaccines where the diseases are inactivated or parts of the disease are used to stimulate an immune response. Thimerosal should never be used in live vaccines, that's because it would kill the microbes you are trying to become immune to due to its cellular toxicity. This, however, creates a new problem and flaw in their logic, your entire body is made of microbes, so the real question should be how could this NOT negatively affect you? People are told that thimerosal is safe by health authorities, but since 1999 the CDC and the American Academy of Pediatrics (AAP) have told manufacturers of vaccines to phase it out. However, it is still an ingredient in many Influenza A and B shots, which is the common cold and we are told to get that shot every year. Think about it, if thimerosal in vaccines were safe why did they backtrack their story and then demand its removal from other vaccines? The sheer disregard for your freedom to choose what you want to go into your body or the body of your child are dwindling by the day and COVID 19 is making it official. Politicians and health officials conveniently talk about the science when they are trying to sell this crap to the masses and yet disregard the science that contradicts their agenda, they cannot have it both ways. America is amongst the worst with Australia not too far behind, by the time a child is 5 they would have had as many as 37 mandatory vaccinations in the US.

Globally it's not much better, here in Australia and many places around the world you cannot send your child to school if they have not been vaccinated and they are now trying to enforce that anyone who hasn't had a vaccination cannot claim unemployment benefits, which says to me that this is only the calm before the storm. With Covid 19 now apparent to everyone in the world they now have the perfect excuse to carry out their controlled crash of the economy and bring in a new monetary system which will abolish cash and make everything digital, trapping and tracking everyone in the system and this has been the plan all along.

If your a pro-vax person then I would like you to keep an open mind on some of the things we are going to look at because soon you will see the truth is anything but what you are told. The question pro-vax people should ask when it comes to people not wanting to vaccinate is, where is the risk to the vaccinated? The whole ideology of getting a vaccine is to prevent disease, so why would the vaccinated be worried by the non vaccinated if that's what they believe? The truth is that many people who are vaccinated get the disease they were being vaccinated for, which raises the question, how safe and effective are vaccinations? Some facts left out by authorities is that vaccines are actually big business and what you're about to learn is what a little research can do before jumping the gun and giving an opinion on a subject you know little about. At least by reading this chapter you can say that you were better informed than before and even if you choose to continue this practice then at least you can say you know the risks. I promise that if you have not done a 180 by the end of this chapter then it will leave you questioning as to why your doctor never told you about these risks before they gave you or your child the shot they say carries no harm. Like GMOs and Flouride the history of vaccines is a mile long and started with a guy called Edward Jenner who is considered to be the father of vaccinology. The first smallpox vaccination was introduced in 1798 after he had inoculated a 13-year-old boy with vaccinia virus (cowpox), which resulted in the boy developing immunity to smallpox, at least that's the official story. Though the concept or idea of vaccination started as a noble one it has morphed into this morally deranged corporate monster backed and protected by government which has prevented anyone from suing a manufacturer of a vaccine no matter what harm it causes. No other product in the world is protected like this and is what I refer to as the protection of corruption. One important fact commonly overlooked or ignored by pro vapers is the decline in mortality from the 1900s to the present day and the year vaccines for certain diseases were introduced. The graph on the next page by the American Academy of Pediatrics shows that some of the major diseases we vaccinate for were already in decline before the vaccines were introduced, meaning that the vaccine is not the reason the disease is gone or in decline.

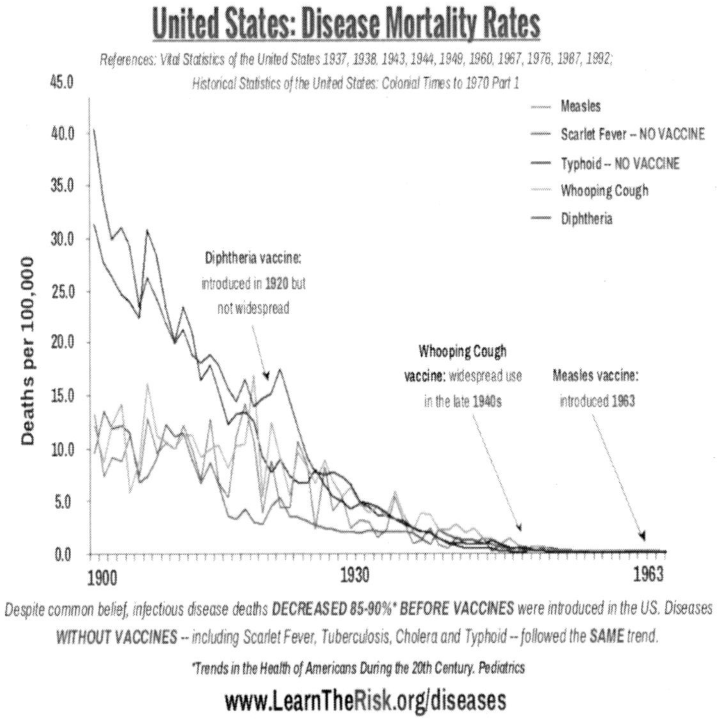

What this does show is that BIG Pharma has hijacked the credit for why these diseases were in decline and have used this information to fuel the fear and success of vaccines worldwide which is projected to make more than 59 billion dollars in the year 2020. With the COVID 19 Scamdemic underway it looks like they may even exceed that figure if people don't start paying attention to what is going on. Another example of diseases that we vaccinate for which were in decline before a vaccine was introduced can be seen in the following graph.

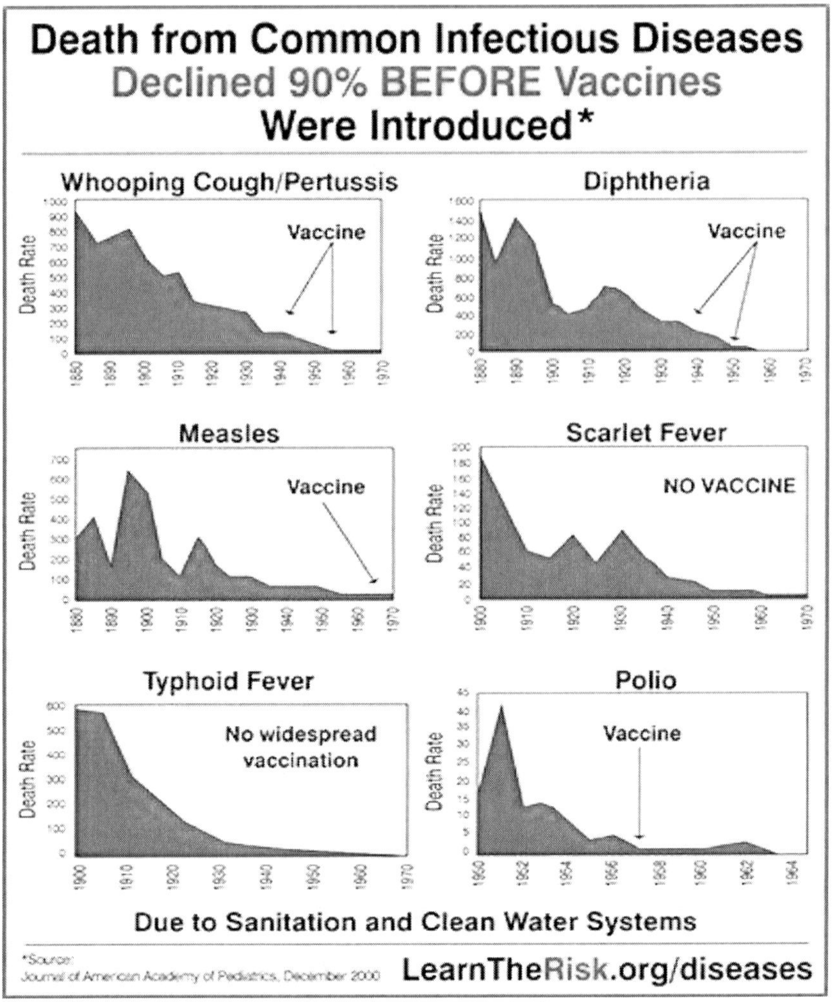

So what is a vaccine? Put simply it is an antigenic substance whereby a piece of the causative agent from the disease (sometimes a synthetic version of it), is injected into you to provide an immune response.

Officially, a successful vaccination is determined by triggering an antigen response; if this occurs then it has fulfilled the official criteria for it to be deemed as an effective vaccine. However, this is a premature assessment, for a vaccine to trigger an autoimmune response it can take months and even years to determine if it is been successful, yet the official follow up period is only 2 weeks. The proof why vaccines are not what they appear to be is seen when someone is vaccinated and gets sick with the disease shortly after. Historically, the cause of many diseases has been due to unsanitary environments, poor nutrition and unclean water, which is still seen in many parts of the world today. If we look at factory farming practices as an example, you'll notice that you have a large concentration of animals in a small amount of space covered in their faeces from head to toe, it's these conditions that are the perfect breeding ground for superbugs and new diseases. This is why so many meat and dairy products are loaded with antibiotics and pain killers otherwise the animals probably wouldn't survive. When we eat these animals we are getting exposed to these drugs used to suppress diseases and it has had a huge impact on our health and our immune system. We have also compounded the problem with our overuse of domestic and commercial cleaners, antibiotics, antiseptic creams, and soaps which have simultaneously lowered our immunity as these superbugs have developed resistance.

The seriousness of this divergence cannot be overstated and one day we are going to see a disease so virulent and deadly that it will make the black plague look like a flea bite on an elephant's ass. Vaccines don't just contain a piece of the disease that you're trying to be immune to they are loaded with toxic and carcinogenic chemicals such as:

Aluminium hydroxide which is a toxic salt, formaldehyde and mercury compounds like thimerasol which are known human carcinogens, they also contain polysorbate 80 which is used as a spermicide in contraception, 2 phenoxyethanol (an Insect repellent), magnesium sulphate (used as fertiliser), sodium chloride, antibiotics, Monosodium Glutamate (MSG) and even aborted fetal tissue and animal proteins from cows, monkeys, chickens, eggs, mice and yeast.

Aluminium is an integral ingredient in most vaccines and studies have shown that when injected 100% of it is absorbed by the body as opposed to dietary aluminium which passes through the kidneys and is flushed out of the body, injectable aluminium can take as long as 8 years to flush out of your body. When aluminium is combined with fluoride which there is an abundance of in tap water it creates a compound called Aluminium tetrafluoride, which is an excellent phosphate mimic which then attaches its self to the receptors in the brain and inhibiting the Adenosine Triphosphate (ATP) which is the production of energy, this may explain in part why so many people feel so tired all the time especially after the doctor has given them one of these toxic cocktails. Aluminium is used in vaccines as an adjuvant, an adjuvant is used to continuously stimulate new antibodies by basically irritating the immune system causing inflammation and damage to the body's tissues. In a study done by the University of British Columbia in Vancouver called *"Aluminium vaccine adjuvants: are they safe"* said the following in their abstract.

Despite almost 90 years of widespread use of aluminium adjuvants, medical science's understanding about their mechanisms of action is still remarkably poor. There is also a concerning scarcity of data on toxicology and pharmacokinetics of these compounds. In spite of this, the notion that aluminium in vaccines is safe appears to be widely accepted. Experimental research, however, clearly shows that aluminium adjuvants have a potential to induce serious immunological disorders in humans.

In particular, aluminium in adjuvant form carries a risk for autoimmunity, long-term brain inflammation and associated neurological complications and may thus have profound and widespread adverse health consequences. In our opinion, the possibility that vaccine benefits may have been overrated and the risk of potential adverse effects underestimated has not been rigorously evaluated in the medical and scientific community. We hope that the present paper will provide a framework for a much needed and long overdue assessment of this highly contentious medical issue.

Information on vaccine ingredients that appear to be widely accepted as mentioned in this study should ring alarm bells and have people in the streets demanding answers from their government about how they justify the continuation of an unscientifically proven practice especially when there is a law protecting it. It is well known within the scientific community that there are no known safety levels of many of the chemicals used in vaccines on adults or even animal studies which should have been the first thing they looked at. Another study called *"Exposure to Mercury and Aluminium in Early Life: Developmental Vulnerability as a Modifying Factor in Neurologic and Immunologic Effects"* by professor José G. Dórea at the Department of Nutrition, Faculty of Health Sciences, Universidade de Brasilia, in Brazil said this in his study:

Currently, ethylmercury (EtHg) and adjuvant-Al are the dominating interventional exposures encountered by fetuses, newborns, and infants due to immunization with Thimerosal-containing vaccines (TCVs). Despite their long use as active agents of medicines and fungicides, the safety levels of these substances have never been determined, either for animals or for adult humans—much less for fetuses, newborns, infants, and children.

Rigorous and replicable studies (in different animal species) have shown evidence of EtHg, and of Al toxicities. More research attention has been given to EtHg and findings have showed a solid link with neurotoxic effects in humans; however, the potential synergic effect of both toxic agents has not been properly studied. Therefore, early life exposure to both EtHg and Al deserves due consideration.

So ask yourself this, if the synergistic effects of the ingredients used in vaccines have never been tested for their safety then how can a doctor tell you a vaccine is safe? We are told as a community that we need to achieve herd immunity which makes a lot of sense if only they weren't destroying it with vaccination. There are 2 types of herd immunity, one called natural herd immunity and the other is apparently achieved through vaccination. Here is how herd immunity works.

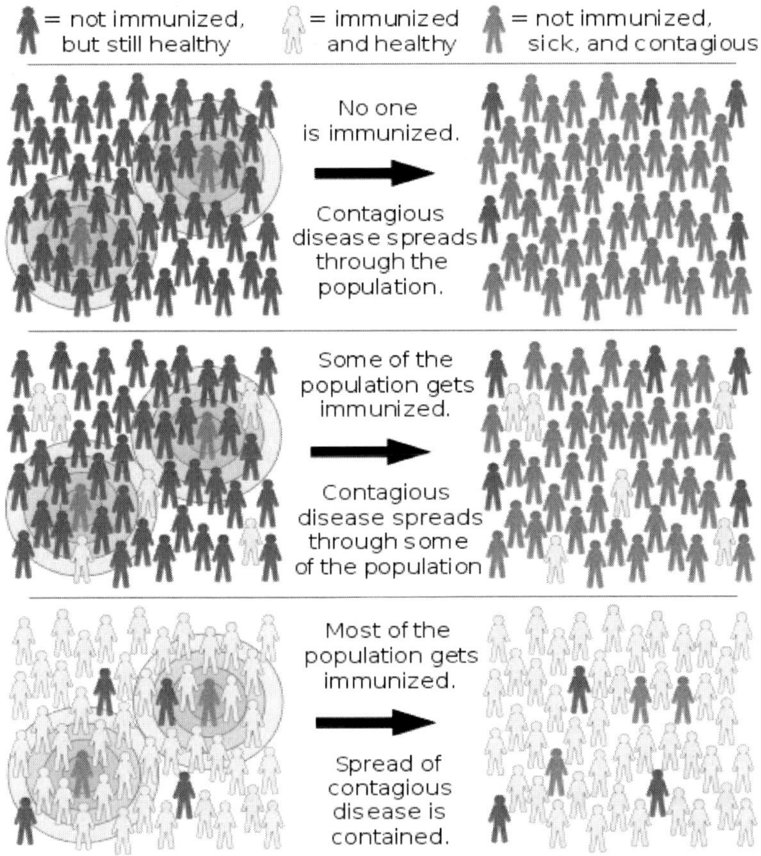

Natural herd immunity happens when the mother of a child is exposed to mild diseases such as chickenpox at a young age and develops antibodies which are then passed on to her children later in life. Because a baby's immune system is underdeveloped, antibodies from the mother are passed on to the child when they are in the mother's womb and through breastfeeding. When a child gets mumps or chickenpox early in life they already have a partial resistance due to the mother's antibodies, which is why they are rarely fatal.

The problem with vaccinations according to Dr Andrew Wakefield, particularly where mumps is concerned, is that vaccination displaces a mild disease early in life to a deadly one the older they get. This is why adults who get mild diseases such as chickenpox and mumps can be fatal the older they are. Another example Dr Wakefield gave is that the chickenpox vaccine which was primarily developed to keep mothers at work made diseases more serious than they needed to be which is why we are now seeing childhood diseases affect people in older demographics worldwide. Vaccines have always been more about money than public health, the annual immunisation cost of a child in 1986 was only $100, yet today it is more than $2,192 per child. This is a staggering increase and with the government mandating more and more vaccinations this is projected to increase well into the future.

Since the 1990's the World Health Organization claims that there are more than 10,000 patent applications each year with the word vaccination in the claim. The World Health Organisation also estimates that by the year 2025 that Big Pharma's profits will reach more than 100 billion dollars which should tell you that Big Pharma is not about disease prevention, it's about pleasing shareholders. As a civilization, we are sicker now than we have ever been and vaccinations are just one of the major problems contributing to this.

In the 1950s the polio vaccine had been contaminated with a monkey virus called Simian Virus 40 (SV40), which has been found in human cancers that affect the brain, bone, mesotheliomas, lymphomas, kidney diseases and even the blood samples of healthy donors. Officially, the Immunization Safety Review Committee established by the Institute of Medicine of the National Academies had concluded that insufficient evidence exists to either accept or reject this claim, which sounds to me like a convenient way to discount any evidence that points to vaccines being the cause of the contamination. Some experts even suggested that evidence points to the monkey virus existing in the human population before the Polio Vaccine was administered. I mean C'mon, Seriously? Who the fuck are these idiots? It is ridiculous to suggest that it is more plausible that humans contracted Simian Virus 40 on this scale by eating, having sex or whatever the mode of contraction was is more probably as opposed to the simplest explanation which is their shitty little-contaminated vaccine doesn't work, and personally find this insulting to our intelligence... Yet the public will believe anything these people say as long as it comes from the TV.

Here is the irony, not only can vaccines cause cancer due to the cancer-causing chemicals they contain but the Human Papilloma Virus Vaccine (HPV) is given to young woman between age of 15 and 25 to prevent cervical cancer. Yet according to Pediatrician Lawrence Palevsky MD, Polysorbate 80 an ingredient in the HPV vaccine is dangerous when combined with other vaccine ingredients because it allows toxic chemicals to pass through the blood-brain barrier which could lead to disorders like Autism and many other neurological conditions, it has also been shown to cause infertility in rat studies.

The documentary "The Greater Good...Think You Know Everything About Vaccines... Think Again", follows the story of a teenage girl called Gabi Swank who got Merck's Gardasil Vaccine Shot, which apparently protects a woman against cervical cancer and how the HPV shot ruined her life leaving her in pain and on more than 40 pills a day to manage her symptoms from what could have been prevented if her parents only knew some of what we have covered here. Vaccines have not only caused many deaths, but they are suspected of being one of the leading causes of Autism which has grown astronomically over the past 30-40 years. It is estimated that in 1990 autism rates in children were 1 in 10,000, but today it's 1 in 68, this is a mind-blowing increase and what do the experts say is the cause? They don't know, but they claim it's not vaccination...

Here is a list of side effects from the adverse event list that have been reported from vaccinations. If you want to learn more than what is listed here then go to the CDC's Vaccine Adverse Event Reporting System. www.vaers.hhs.gov.

Mild Reactions

Dizziness, rashes, coughs, nausea, anger/rage, irritability, emotional distress.

Severe Reactions

Brachial neuritis, cerebrovascular accident (stroke), chronic rheumatoid arthritis, convulsions, seizures, febrile seizure, death, encephalopathy and encephalitis (brain swelling), hearing loss, Guillain-Barré syndrome, immune system disorders, lymphatic system disorders, multiple sclerosis, myocarditis, nervous system disorders, neurological syndromes including autism, pain in extremity, paralysis and myelitis including transverse myelitis, peripheral neuropathy, pneumonia and lower respiratory infections, skin and tissue disorders including eczema, sudden infant death syndrome

(SIDS), tinnitus (ringing in the ears), vaccine-strain versions of chickenpox, measles, mumps, polio, influenza, meningitis, yellow fever, and pertussis, vasculitis (inflammation of blood vessels).

Parents who have vaccinated their children where an adverse event takes place have often said that they have watched their children crash within hours, and these parents are constantly haunted by their decision to vaccinate because they were not told of the risks! Lives have been ruined and families ripped apart as an unwavering sadness overwhelms these parents because THEY signed the consent form and THEY held their child down while the doctor gave it to them. When an adverse event takes place and the vaccination is suspected of being the cause doctors will deny its involvement and simply tell you that your child must have had a previously undiagnosed condition, there is zero accountability.

Another thing your doctor won't tell you is that until recently there had never been a safety or effectiveness study on vaccinated vs unvaccinated, can you believe that! The study is called "*Pilot comparative study on the health of vaccinated and unvaccinated 6-to 12-year old U.S. children*" by Professor Anthony R Mawson at the Department of Epidemiology and Biostatistics, School of Public Health, Jackson State University, Jackson, USA. The study looked at children who were homeschooled which had a higher rate of being unvaccinated compared to those in public schooling. The study showed that unvaccinated children had a higher risk of getting chickenpox and pertussis which is whooping cough and considered to be a mild disease, but were less likely to develop pneumonia, otitis media (middle ear infections), allergies and neurodegenerative disorders. In summary, the study concluded the following in their abstract...

> *In conclusion, vaccinated homeschool children were found to have a higher rate of allergies and Neuro Developmental Disorders (NDD) than unvaccinated homeschool children. While vaccination remained significantly associated with NDD after controlling for other factors, preterm birth coupled with vaccination was associated with an apparent synergistic increase in the odds of NDD. Further research involving larger, independent samples and stronger research designs is needed to verify and understand these unexpected findings in order to optimize the impact of vaccines on children's health.*

According to Dr Andrew Wakefield, this study went through at least 4 rounds of peer review before being published because of how controversial the subject was, which tells you that some journals are only interested in maintaining the narrative and not real science. If anything, it might encourage the CDC and other health authorities to get off their ass and do their job in the interest of public health and safety. This study received a lot of criticism from the public, but if you read it plainly and not try to interpret it like the bible or the Koran, it clearly says in the conclusion that further research is needed. I have nothing but respect for Professor Mawson because he dared to question and put his career on the line doing what the CDC and other government health departments should have done from the beginning, and that to me is what counts.

One of the authorities selling this crap to the public is American paediatrician Paul Offit, who is the Chief of Infectious Diseases and the Director of the Vaccine Education Centre at the Children's Hospital of Philadelphia (CHOP). He is also credited with saying what I believe was the most reckless, dangerous and stupid thing to ever leave a human beings mouth on vaccine safety, and that was, "A baby's immune system could handle as many as 10,000 vaccines". He actually said that and even pro-vaxers thought that was a bit much so what does that tell you? That's like me saying if I hit him over the head 10,000 times with a copy of my book then he might learn something from it. As eager as I would be to put that into practice I don't see him subjecting himself to 10,000 injections of the rotavirus he created and sold to Merck for 186 million dollars, of which he got approximately 29 million, so it's no wonder he told a whole nation this, he had 29 million reasons to say it. The worst part is that other doctors listen to this guy because he is considered to be an authority on the subject. Paul Offit is also a consultant for the pharmaceutical company Merck who funded his research at CHOP in 1998, but more shockingly he sat at the US CDC advisory board which makes decisions about public health issues and contributes to the approval of certain drugs and vaccines along with the FDA to be used in the public domain. But it gets worse, the FDA and the CDC do not enforce conflict of interest rules, so anyone who holds a patent or stock for any drug or vaccine, which everyone on the advisory board does, can approve it even if it's unsafe or is dangerous and without consequence! Everyone on the advisory board at the CDC has an invested interest of some kind, and that's not me saying this, this is what the Inspector General of the US health and Human Services (HHS) said.

The pharmaceutical industry has spent more money than Oil and Insurance on lobbying for favourable laws to get vaccines and other drugs they manufacturer fast-tracked and into the market place. When the department of health approves a vaccines use the safety trial on the drug is dropped because it is assumed to be safe, like this COVID 19 jab they a rushed through. This is another reason why we do not have any long term safety studies on vaccinated vs unvaccinated or their effectiveness. This is exactly how medications can pass with government approval only to later be recalled when the long term use of the drug is found to produce side effects. Vaccines are not about science they are about politics, power, marketing and money, all designed to convince the masses that you need what they sell.

According to Robert F Kennedy Jr. who is an American radio host, environmental activist, author and attorney specializing in environmental law, the CDC itself is a VACCINE COMPANY, with patents to 20 vaccines making more than 4.1 billion dollars every year. It's no wonder you have people like Paul Offit going on national television saying the rubbish he does. I bet he doesn't know that there is enough mercury in a silver filling to force the shutdown of a 10-acre lake, if you had 10,000 vaccinations with thimerasol alone then it boggles the mind to think how many people it could kill.

In a YouTube video of congressmen, Dan Bourke in the US he clearly stated that his grandson was given 9 vaccinations in one hit and 7 of them had thimerasol, a couple of days later he was autistic. You cannot have so many people saying the same thing without there being something to it, it goes way beyond just coincidence!

We must open our eyes to vaccinations and see them for what they are, historically man has gotten over some of the worst diseases imaginable and we did it without vaccinations. Some examples are, yellow fever, scurvy, smallpox, scarlet fever, tuberculosis and the even the bubonic plague which happened between 1348 to 1350 in Europe and killed more than 25 million people, that's a death rate of 30-50% which today would be 370,500,000 people. So why don't we see these diseases all over the place today? I'm not saying that they don't exist still, I'm simply making the point that we don't have a vaccine for them and yet they are no longer threats to our society. The truth is that we did something better than vaccination, we addressed the root cause of the problem by improving our standards of living which included better sanitary practices and cleaner living environments.

The Graph below shows TB rates in decline in the US

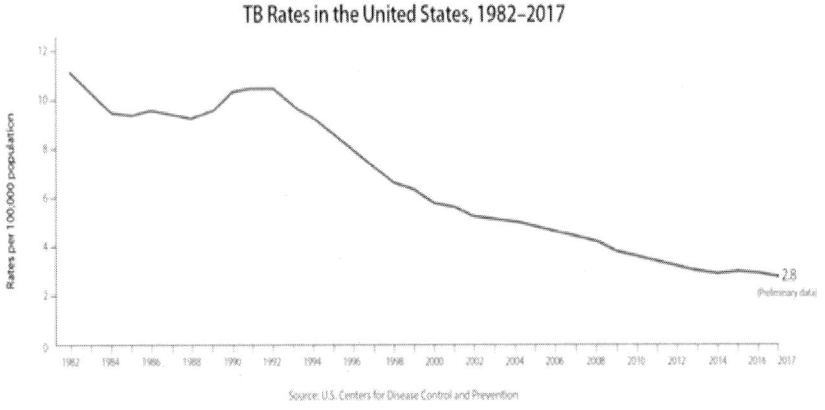

This chart is from the CDC's website and they admit that the BCG vaccine used for TB is not widely given to people in the US and it doesn't always work. So if people don't normally get the vaccine and it doesn't always work why is TB in decline?

Another example is Scarlet fever, which is a bacterial infection caused by group A Streptococcus, the CDC admits that it is a mild disease commonly see in children up to 15 years of age, but can affect any age group and yet in the mid-19th century it was considered to be one of the deadliest diseases in England which in some parts had a fatality rate of 30%. Today you pop a few antibiotics and you're on your way, no vaccine fixed this issue. According to the CDC, around 300 deaths occur each year due to Typhoid Fever, it is caused when a person eats food or drinks water with faeces by an infected person. Worldwide it is estimated that 22 million cases of typhoid are seen each year where approximately 200,000 of them will die. This is one of my favourite examples of how a vaccine is not needed to fix Typhoid Fever because the solution to the problem is for people not to eat or drink their own shit! Obviously, the solution is better water treatment protocols, waste management and food handling. Many of those in the US that get typhoid fever have travelled overseas, its a very preventable disease should the right infrastructure and water treatment facilities be in place.

We have eliminated the majority of the black plague by improving our living standards and it wasn't a vaccine that saved us, we know this because it occurred in the 1300s whereas the first vaccine didn't appear till 1796, more than 450 years later. How are we to evolve as a species if we are so afraid of ridicule for actually speaking our minds and asking the tough questions authorities don't want us asking? It's obvious to anyone who bothers to look that we don't have all the answers, so before mindlessly subjecting future generations to this practice we need clarity on what we are doing.

What I have shared here is just a fraction of the whole story, so before you get your next flu shot or subject your child to another vaccination take 1 hour of your time and research the opposite of what you believe and see if it makes sense to you. If you're an X-files fan then you'll know that Deep throat said it best, "a lie is most convincingly hidden between two truths", and I absolutely believe that.

Ultimately, I have tried to make this book the canary in the coal mine because for most of us the damage of vaccines is not always evident, it's no different to not being able to taste fluoride in the water or see or smell the chemicals in GMO's, like in a coal mine, just because you cannot see, taste, smell or touch poisonous gas doesn't mean it's not there. Developing a healthy awareness about vaccinations will make a world of difference to whether you get cancer or other chronic illnesses. Only a few years ago my mother had always been an advocate of vaccination but now she refuses to get any, she also works in a hospital so you would think she would get sick all the time, but she is lucky if she gets a common cold once a year. Only recently my grandfather had a flu shot recommended by his doctor and even though I told him not to do it, being old and stubborn seemed to take precedence. A couple of days after he got pneumonia and was bedridden for nearly a month, a week of which was spent in the hospital, now even he suspects that it was the flu shot that did it to him. This may seem like a biased view on this subject but the truth is that there are people all over the world experiencing exactly what I just described with my family.

Today the common cold is hitting people hard and many young people are even dying. This is another contradiction in vaccination because every year we are told by doctors and the media to get our flu shots, but if most people are getting them then why is the flu so bad? So take a moment to ask the question, is it possible that some of the things you have learned so far could be causing your illness? Since the beginning of time nature had already worked out what was needed to make humans healthy, are we so arrogant to think that we need to improve upon something that is not broken? You are more powerful than you realize and your freedom to choose what goes in your body is not a privilege, it's a basic human right, one that should be viciously defended.

If you want to find the ingredients and the manufacturer of a vaccine then visit www.procon.org. For further research I would recommend the documentary Vaxxed which was considered to be an anti-vax documentary and received a lot of criticism, it is not the only documentary out there, so all I can say is the more you learn the better informed you will be.

CHAPTER 11: 7 THINGS THAT ARE MAKING YOU WORSE

So far we have covered GMO's, fluoride and vaccines, which should help you better understand the risks of the food, water and medications you are taking and see them in a new light. Here we will look at 7 other things that are making your cancer worse and by eliminating as many of these as possible you are setting yourself up for the best results. We will now take a look at how sugar, meat, dairy, smoking, alcohol, medications and how even your attitude can affect your overall health and wellbeing.

When my father's cancer returned surgery wasn't an option and they were recommending chemotherapy as their drug of choice. After ignoring my advice he proceeded with the treatment leaving him weak, bedridden and physically unable for at least a week. Of the 7 things this chapter covers he was taking 5 of them where dairy was the exception due to lactose intolerance and he was on no medications aside from the treatment itself. The hospital dietician told him to eat anything he could stomach, her focus was for him to put on more weight so he would handle the chemotherapy better even though eating the junk she mentioned would make his cancer worse. Soon after he was eating everything he shouldn't, coke, ice cream, pies and pizza all loaded with sugar. He had a range of symptoms from the treatment including insomnia, irritability, burning sensations, memory problems, nausea and concentration problems which is called chemo brain.

During the second round of treatment I heard him get up one night when a loud bang suddenly got me on my feet, he had collapsed against the wall gashing his head and lying on the floor.

My mother was freaking out and thanks to my sister being more level headed than my mother, called the ambulance and described what had happened. The ambulance arrived and he was immediately taken to Box Hill hospital, after a few tests it was determined that his blood pressure was extremely low which caused the fainting. It wasn't until later that we discovered that he should never have had the chemo treatment with his blood pressure so low. We knew this was the cause because when I took him no one had bothered to check it before giving the treatment to him. This is the kind of incompetence you can expect from hospitals and it is no exaggeration in saying that these people will kill you if you don't stay vigilant.

When I visited him the next day with my mother and sister I noticed something when I looked at the daily menu for him, everything on it was sugar and processed foods. It actually blew my mind at the kind of food doctors let cancer patients have when they know better than anyone the role sugar plays in cancer growth. This was when I first found out that cancer patients who are hospitalised are not on controlled diets and even the dieticians have no idea about the role these foods play in cancer growth. After googling a few key words I soon found that many other people including doctors were asking the same questions and having the same concerns as I were, proving to me that this was not an overreaction.

So let's begin this chapter with sugar because it's our favourite poison and it's absolutely critical that you understand how your cancer responds to it.

SUGAR

Today sugar is in just about everything especially products where it says 99% fat-free, what they don't tell you is that they doubled the sugar because 99% fat-free means it tastes like crap and therefore it won't sell. Food companies know exactly how to market their products to people, especially to children, putting their favourite cartoon characters on all sorts of products including fast food. What these companies don't say is how addictive and damaging sugar is for the body and the mind, its effects even rival that of alcohol and drugs.

Sugar is a term describing a class of molecules called carbohydrates, anytime you buy a product with Glucose, Fructose, Sucrose, Maltose, Lactose, Dextrose and starch you are talking about sugar. A study done by Dr Nicole Avena of the Icahn School of Medicine at Mount Sinai said that pizza is the most addictive food by far because of the sugar found in the tomato sauce and that one slice had more sugar than a couple of Oreos. This revelation was a major blow for me because I love my pizza, it also reflected other studies I read showing how highly palatable processed foods can change human behaviour by altering brain your chemistry to show the same changes seen in addiction from alcoholics and drug addicts. Sugar is also 8 times more addictive than cocaine, a study done with 43 mice showed that 40 out of 43 preferred sugar water to cocaine water, cocaine is also known to be one of the hardest drugs to quit. Sugar has this effect by hijacking your brain by telling your body that you are hungry even when your stomach is full. People actually believe that they are making their own choices about what they eat, but they are dead wrong, chemical influence is dictating over behavioural choice and these food companies exploit this like you wouldn't believe.

To better understand how the brain works we can make a comparison between a vegetable like broccoli and a chocolate cupcake, 9/10 will go for the cupcake, I would go for the cupcake, this is because our brains have evolved to go for the foods which have the highest calorie intake. Before this big bang of junk food, it wasn't so easy to come by, in our hunter-gatherer days most people had to get what they could while they could get it. In the 21st century where the only calories you burn is by picking up the phone to call the pizza guy, it's no wonder people are obese and have all these diseases and disorders. It also explains why children go bat shit crazy after drinking things like coke or red cordial, their brains are being hijacked and are exhibiting the same behaviour seen in addicts. The average person consumes approximately 32 teaspoons of sugar every day where high-fructose corn syrup makes up 8, corn syrup is in so many products it boggles the mind, the daily recommended amount of sugar is 6-9 teaspoons where the total consumption works out to be nearly 30 pounds of sugar every year.

A study done by neuroscientist Fernando Gomez-Pinilla at the University of California Los Angeles showed that sweet drinks make rats stupid and inhibit learning and memory. First, the scientists trained all of the rats to successfully navigate a maze, then they divided the group in two, giving one half a controlled diet and the other a fructose syrup diet which made up 15%. After 6 weeks it was shown the high fructose diet took the group 30% longer to complete the maze than the control group. The rat's brains were also dissected and it was found that a high fructose diet had caused the synapses in the brain to change, a process essential to learning, it also showed to affect the hippocampus which is an area in the brain that works the same in humans for memory formation.

Too much sugar has also been shown to cause the following:

Alzheimer's, diabetes, obesity, heart disease, suppresses the immune system, non-alcoholic liver disease, raises your cholesterol, chromium deficiency, hypoglycaemia, arthritis, appendicitis, kidney damage, liver damage, oxidative stress, depression, crankiness in children, and potentially cause cancer and make it significantly worse for those who already have it.

So you might be wondering what exactly is sugars role in cancer? Sugar is cancers PRIMARY fuel source, it causes inflammation and makes the blood more acidic creating the conditions it needs to grow. This acidity is not to be confused with the acidity of your gut, your gut should be highly acidic to break down foods properly, but the blood should have a ph range of 7.2-7.5. Cancers metabolic rate is faster than that of healthy cells so you can starve your cancer by reducing or eliminating your sugar intake. This is important to remember! If you change the conditions of your cancer from an acidic to an alkaline environment then cancer won't grow! That's because in an acidic environment oxygen is deprived and oxygen is poisonous to cancer cells.

Sugar has had an enormous impact on human health and what we call food today, go back as little as 50 years and our relationship with sugar was very different. Traditional methods of preserving and processing like salting, curing, curdling, drying, pickling and smoking never had such health risks associated with them and having more salt in the diet is exactly what is needed not less.

It was only since the 19th century and the industrial revolution that food manufacturing was born and what led to this over-consumption of processed foods which have nutritionally deprived most people today. We have become detached from our roots and have morphed into this mindless synthetic monster to line the pockets of our enslavers at the expense of our health. We need to rediscover traditional techniques that do not carry such consequences to our health and improve our relationship with sugar which has become one of abuse. This is why so many people addicted to food find it impossible to quit when they are surrounded by it all the time. Is it reasonable to tell an alcoholic to quit if you put them in a bottle shop? Of course not! How is it any different to quit or cut back your sugar intake when you are constantly bombarded with advertising and marketing hijacking your brain telling you to eat more? As long as corporations are allowed to manipulate and abuse our relationship with sugar our problems will continue, these companies even tell us that they are not responsible because the government sets the standards on what's allowed. This is a total cop-out because these companies pay governments handsomely for their favourable laws so why would they stop? It is no different to a drug dealer saying it's your fault you're addicted to drugs even though the addiction occurred because the dealer made it available to the addict.

Sugar is a double-edged sword, it is essential for cellular function but it's where we get our sugar from that's important, like the difference between a teaspoon of processed white sugar or from a punnet of strawberries. Natural sources are the best because they contain fibre, which means it takes longer for the sugar to be used and does not tell our pancreas to produce fat right away. I often liken cancer patients to pregnant women in the sense that when they try to improve their diet, strong cravings will try to overcome them. This is the bad bacteria in the gut and cancer releasing chemicals which hijacks the brain telling them you to eat more high sugar foods so it can grow. These bad gut bacteria can be controlled better with a broad-spectrum probiotic which can reduce the cravings, combined with a B vitamin complex supplement and you will feel fuller longer without the craving for high sugar foods.

Believe it or not, doctors have known about sugars role in cancer for more than 100 years thanks to a guy called Dr Otto Heinrich Warburg who was a German physiologist, medical doctor and won the Nobel Prize in 1931 for the discovery of the nature and mode of action of the respiratory enzyme. His work concentrated on how a cancer cell uses energy and was the first to show that cancer cells use sugar faster than normal cells. Yet doctors today do not warn you about the role sugar plays in your diet after being diagnosed which is nothing short of false, misleading and deceptive.

In a Ted X talk called "Starving Cancer Away" by Dr Sophia Lunt at Michigan State University, she talks about the relationship cancer and sugar has with our cells and also the differences between a normal cell and a cancer cell. In the presentation, Dr Lunt makes an interesting point that unlike our normal cells which have a fixed way of metabolizing in our bodies, cancer cells can alter their metabolism. This means that if a particular treatment tries to kill cancer in only one way cancer will adapt to find another way to get what it needs to grow. This may also explain why the one size fits all approach oncologists use to treat patients has a low success rate. It is also validating in what people who take that natural approach say by simultaneously starving cancer by depriving it of sugar while increasing their intake of anti-cancer foods that attack cancer and boost the immune system.

There are hundreds if not thousands of studies on sugar and how it can impact your health, so while you are recovering sugar and processed foods like bread's, pasta's and cereals are to be avoided. Furthermore, try to avoid potatoes and sweet potatoes and focus more on organic vegetables that have a high nutrient content relative to their sugars.

DAIRY

I used to love milk, love it! But after learning what goes into it let's just say I have developed a healthy awareness towards this family favourite at breakfast time and have switched to healthier alternatives. Most people know that milk has hormones in it, bovine hormones called bGH, rbGH, and bST, which is given to cows to make them mature faster and to produce more milk. But milk has so much more than just these hormones and whether you have cancer or not you may want to rethink what you are putting in your coffee and giving your children at breakfast time.

Dairy has been linked to a whole range of medical conditions such as acne which is a result of elevated insulin levels by the insulin growth factor hormone (IG1) found in all dairy, it can also give people mood swings because of the excess estrogen and testosterone which get out of balance. The hormones in milk are so high that they even exceed the level of hormones in the female cow during impregnation. According to Dr Epstein, Professor of Environmental and Occupational Medicine at the University of Illinois School of Public Health, and Chairman of the Cancer Prevention Coalition, the recombinant Bovine Growth Hormone (rBGH) amplifies the level of IGF-1 hormone which increases the risk of breast, colon and prostate cancer. Cows that are injected with this hormone are done so in times when they should not be feeding calves, instead, it forces them to produce milk all year round for increased productivity.

The rBGH hormone is manmade and once given to a cow they are prone to regular infections which creates puss in the milk causing it to turn sour, this is then combated by giving the cow more and more antibiotics to keep the milk from spoiling. Aside from hormones and antibiotics here are some other things found in Pasteurised milk:

- Niflumic acid – anti-inflammatory/painkiller
- Mefenamic acid – anti-inflammatory
- Flunixin – anti-inflammatory
- Ibuprofen – painkiller
- Diclofenac – anti-inflammatory
- Ketoprofen – anti-inflammatory
- Florfenicol – antibiotic
- 17B-estradiol – sex hormone
- Triclosan – anti-fungal drug
- Pyrimethamine – anti-malaria drug
- 17a-ethinylestradiol – steroid hormone

For cows to get regular infections just to keep them productive all year round sounds to me like we have some very sick cows producing our milk, and it's a no-brainer that sick cows lead to sick people. The saying you are what you eat is not quite accurate, you are what you eat eats if that makes sense. Just from a welfare point of view look at how many painkillers are being used, exactly how much pain are these animals in? What are the side effects of humans consuming milk with all these nasty drugs?

If so many drugs are being used in the production of normal milk why are consumers not made aware of what they are drinking? 99% of people have no idea what they are drinking and I bet if they did they would make different health choices hurting the dairy industries bank balance. These effects become more obvious particularly where children are concerned; a young developing child does not need hormones in their food which can have a whole range of adverse side effects in their developing years. Dairy has also been linked to diabetes, autoimmune disorders, schizophrenia and multiple sclerosis, the countries with the highest dairy consumption also have the highest rate of osteoporosis.

Experts could debate the risks of pasteurized vs unpasteurized milk till the cows come home, but logically it makes sense that historically farmers who never pasteurized their milk or stuffed them full of chemicals lived long and healthy lives otherwise many of us wouldn't be here. I would argue that traditional farming practices were amongst the healthiest and safest when done properly to both animal and human. In the old days we didn't factory farm or inject cows with hormones to trick their bodies into calving 12 month's at a time, nor did we have these ridiculous laws that say we have to stuff perfectly healthy cows full of chemicals just to sell a product so the battling farmer can make a decent living.

In Australia and many parts of the world, it is illegal to sell or give unpasteurized milk to anyone other than your immediate family, the risk is that bacteria on the teat of the cow if not sterilized properly can cause an infection which can be fatal. However, safer practices on the sterilization of the teat of the cow should be their primary concern if that is the greatest risk of unpasteurized milk. The fact that you can buy organic milk where none of these drugs is used is proof that it can be done, unlike the milk most people drink which are from dozy cows that are just as drugged up as they are. This is what happens when you put cows into factory farm environment standing in pens so small they cannot move while feeding them their drug enriched GMO grains all in the name of productivity. The only reason this madness is allowed is that consumers don't want to pay an extra $2 at the supermarket for proper milk and put these people out of business. Then, the same people wonder why they or members of their family are sick! We have done it to ourselves. It's not rocket science, sick animals equal sick people it's a simple equation, you don't need a master degree or some expert wanker on TV trying to explain it to you!

If you have cancer and are trying to recover all dairy is to be avoided completely, if not for the sugar content and the hormone factors then for the medications used in treating the cow's illness while producing milk. In a study called *"Bovine leukaemia virus discovered in human blood"* by Professor

Gertrude Case Buehring at the School of Public Health, the University of California in the USA the study mentioned the following:

Bovine leukemia virus (BLV) infection is widespread in cattle globally and is present in marketed beef and dairy products. Human infection with BLV has been reported in breast and lung cancer tissues and was significantly associated with breast cancer in 3 case-control studies.

The purpose of this current research was to determine if BLV is present in human blood cells and if antibodies to BLV are related to blood cell infection.

This first report of BLV in human blood raises the question of whether infection of leukocytes could conceivably lead to leukemia as it does in infected cattle. Also, system wide circulation of infected blood cells could facilitate BLV transit to various internal tissues/organs with potential for their infection and subsequent development of cancer. The most likely route of BLV transmission to humans would be zoonotic, as a foodborne infection. Although eradicated from cattle in some countries, BLV still has a high rate of infection in the Americas, the Middle East, and parts of Europe and Asia. This report of BLV in the blood layer containing human leukocytes/platelets adds important information which could be useful to elucidate possible routes of transmission of BLV to humans and to prevent further human infection.

Closer to home, Professor Gertrude Case Buehring in Australia was part of another study called *"Bovine leukaemia virus linked to breast cancer in Australian women and identified before breast cancer development"* concluded this in the study:

> *Bovine leukemia virus is significantly associated with breast cancer in a population of Australian women, and was present in some breast tissues 3–10 years before the cancer was diagnosed.*

The criteria for organic milk in Australia is that it must come from a cow and cannot have been treated with any antibiotics or hormones in its growth or reproduction. However vaccines are to be used only when necessary and must be non-GM, antibiotics can be used in emergencies for disease and animal welfare but its milk cannot be sold for 6 months, the cows must be free-range and have access to pasture their whole lives and 5% chemical-free non-organic feed can be used where absolutely necessary. For an extra $2 I'd say you are getting a whole lot for your money compared to the cheap drug-infested milk that is likely to cause hormone imbalances in children and many chronic diseases later in life. Despite knowing these health issues supermarkets seem intent on selling consumers shit while bankrupting good hard-working Aussie farmers. The real question should be, why isn't organic the standard for how all milk is produced? The human digestive system was not designed to break down dairy, in fact, as much as 75% of the world's population is lactose intolerant. What most people don't realise is that if you need calcium in your diet then you don't need a glass of milk, most green leafy vegetables like kale, spinach, or broccoli, are a superior sources of calcium than any dairy product. I love dairy just as much as the rest of us but until safer and healthier practices for both animal and human are evident I'd advise to minimise your intake and always buy organic if you can get it. If you are recovering from cancer, then stay away from it completely until you have recovered, think of it more as a treat and not a go-to snack whenever you get hungry or thirsty.

If you absolutely must have milk then try substituting dairy for organic almond or coconut milk which are healthier alternatives with less sugar. Coconut milk and mixed organic berries are nutrient-dense, sweet to the taste and filling, so try this if you want to satisfy your sweet tooth.

It's important to know that I'm not trying to scare you out of everything in your fridge, but you do need to understand exactly what is in your food because it's obvious that the authorities won't tell you.

MEAT

I love meat as much as the next person but unfortunately, there isn't much room for this in the recovering cancer diet, meat does have a place but it's extremely limited for reasons we will explore. Every natural or alternative treatment I have researched has had one consistent theme and that is to eliminate sugar, dairy and meat from the diet and when you take a closer look at what is used in our meat it's no surprise. Whether you believe it or not meat is full of hormones as we covered in the section on dairy, it's also loaded with that red crap they use to make meat look fresh, oh you didn't know? It's called carbon monoxide, the same carbon monoxide which is found in car exhaust fumes, cigarettes, gas stoves, water heaters, clothes dryers and a ton more. Carbon monoxide can make meat appear red for up to a year and in the US it is estimated that more than 50,000 carbon monoxides poisonings occur each year where symptoms could be anything from headache and cough to coma or death. One interesting and all too familiar characteristic of carbon monoxide is that it is a colourless, odourless and tasteless gas, which sounds a lot like fluoride and all the other chemicals we have covered so far. Carbon monoxide is known for depleting oxygen which can leave people short on breath and in a state of fatigue, in the body it causes inflammation, free radical damage and negatively impacts mitochondrial respiration which is the energy centre of a cell, it also specifically affects the brain and the heart. If carbon monoxide is so great in meat then why is it being banned in most parts of Europe alongside GMOs and Fluoride in their water? Treatment of this type of poisoning is usually hyperbaric oxygen treatment but depending on the severity of exposure treatment is limited.

When beef ages it usually goes brown or greyish, so naturally or should I say unnaturally, it's stuffed full of chemicals to make it look fresher than it is so it's appealing to the consumer. It is also loaded with ammonia to prevent E.coli and bacterial growth and if you read this far I don't need to tell exactly what that can do. A huge study published in the Journal of The National Cancer Institute in 2005 called *"Meat, fish, and colorectal cancer risk: the European Prospective Investigation into Cancer and nutrition,"* which included 10 European countries and 478,040 men and woman that were cancer-free between the years of 1992 to 1998. They concluded that after a mean follow-up of 4.8 years, 1329 people had colorectal cancer which they concluded was positively attributed to high consumption of red and processed meat where people consumed between 20g-160g per day, the study showed that fish had the opposite effect.

Not only is red meat bad for you but the lifestyle that factory-farmed animals are subjected to is totally diabolical, which is why all meats nowadays are loaded with antibiotics and other medications. If you have ever watched a factory farming documentary then you know exactly what I am talking about, it could put you off meat for life, and after watching the last one I went vegetarian for about 3 months. I'm not going to fluff it up by saying it was easy to quit meat especially growing up as I did where every meal is a meat meal. Since then I have done my best to limit how much meat I eat each week and try to buy organic or grass-fed as my budget allows. However, for the recovering cancer patient, the only exception would be wild-caught meats where no chemicals or drugs have been used, your new philosophy on meat while your recovering must be less is more. I strongly believe that if we treated the animals that we consume better and they lived healthier and happier lives as nature intended then there would be far less concern regarding meat, but sadly that is a battle for another day.

Most people don't want to acknowledge how or where our meat comes from. These kinds of people refuse to see animals treated as poorly as they are in a factory farm environment as long as they can get their favourite hamburger from McDonald's at 5:00 am because they were up all night celebrating how oblivious to the world they have become. People like this lack all respect for the sanctity of life and children should be shown exactly what happens to these animals we eat so when parents see the horror in their children's faces they will realise just how wrong this whole process has become.

If livestock were raised on an organic diet with little if any chemical intervention then meat at your supermarket would not be as toxic as it is today, even to healthy people meat poses risks because like everything else mentioned in this book it's just a matter of time before symptoms manifest. There have been many studies on the links between cancer and red meat which show that the risks lye not in the meat itself but the chemicals use to extend its shelf life. Traditional farming and butchers never used such harmful chemicals to extend the shelf life of meat products, if the methods they used back then were so bad then we would have seen similar health issues the further back we go.

I am not the biggest fan of the Cancer Council Australia but even they say on their website that the World Health Organization officially classifies processed meats like ham, bacon, salami and frankfurts as a Group 1 carcinogen, that's the same ranking as arsenic, asbestos, formaldehyde, diesel fuel, plutonium, alcohol, tobacco, hepatitis B & C and even gamma radiation. So why the fuck can you still buy these products at the supermarket without being told the risks? Red meats like beef, lamb and pork are classified as Group 2A, which means that it probably causes cancer to humans, that's only one step down from Group 1.

If you are a meat-eater like myself then I highly recommend going with an experienced hunter for game, if you are killing an animal for food and performing the act yourself will get an entirely new perspective and respect on what a valuable resource these animals are and that protecting and respecting them is the only way forward. If you absolutely must eat red meat then the healthiest I can suggest is that from a proper organic farm or wild-caught meats. As an alternative try paying a hunter a to get a buck or wild goat for your freezer which is a great alternative and a way to keep pest species in check.

Corporations have conditioned society into thinking that meat comes from the supermarket which is why this resource continues to be abused. We are teaching the younger generation to be a bunch of self-entitled spoilt little shits in need of a foot in the ass, particularly the millennials. At the rate we are abusing the limited resources we have on this planet there will come a day not too far in the future when the only time you or your children will see the diversity of life on this planet we have today will be in a picture or the zoo due to this type of livestock raising and that is the greatest crime of all.

SMOKING

I won't go into too much detail here because this is a bit of a no-brainer, but I will chuck a few facts your way in case you didn't know. We all know that smoking can cause cancer and not just lung cancer but cancer of the *nose, mouth, larynx (voice box), trachea, oesophagus, stomach, pancreas, kidneys, bladder, cervix, bone marrow and blood.*

According to the American Lung Association, there are more than 600 ingredients in a cigarette and it produces more than 7000 chemicals while it is burning, 69 of these are known to be carcinogenic.

Here is a short list of the ones mentioned on their website:

- Acetone - found in nail polish remover
- Acetic acid - an ingredient in hair dye
- Ammonia - a common household cleaner
- Arsenic - used in rat poison
- Benzene - found in rubber cement and gasoline
- Butane - used in lighter fluid
- Cadmium - active component in battery acid
- Carbon monoxide - released in car exhaust fumes
- Formaldehyde - embalming fluid
- Hexamine - found in barbecue lighter fluid
- Lead - used in batteries
- Naphthalene - an ingredient in mothballs
- Methanol - a main component in rocket fuel,
- Nicotine - used as an insecticide
- Tar - material for paving roads
- Toluene - used to manufacture paint

When quitting smoking it's important to view it as a lifestyle change rather than a fad or something you feel forced to do due to your condition, your body has probably been telling you for a long time to stop what you are doing and that something wasn't quite right. Believe it or not, smoking is as addictive as heroin and like heroin, it is just as hard to quit, yet it is essential to a speedier recovery if you are tackling cancer, you simply cannot put 7,000 toxic chemicals into your body and expect to be ok, that is not realistic or practical to your recovering efforts. Smoking is also one of the world's leading causes of premature deaths and also one of the most preventable, it accounts for more than 6 million deaths every year worldwide and is expected to go to 8 million by 2030. Smoking can also cause the following:

Infertility, diabetes, increases premature ageing, increases stress levels, poor blood flow, heart disease, lung disease, clotting problems, high cholesterol, problems in newborns, erectile dysfunction and many more.

Despite what some believe passive smoke is just as bad as smoking itself, for example, in the UK it is estimated that more than 10,000 people die from passive smoking every year which is another reason why even if the person who has cancer doesn't smoke that those who do smoke do it somewhere else. Both of my parents had always been smokers and as a kid, I used to lecture them about it all the time, when I told friends that my father got lung cancer the first they said to me was does he smoke? I said yes, but the truth is that smoking isn't the only cause of lung cancer and those who don't smoke can just as easily get it, it was just simpler to say what I did because I didn't want a debate on the subject. Ultimately, it is your choice what you do and the last thing you need to read is a lecture on your lifestyle choices, it will only drive you to smoke more because you already know something is wrong. The information here is to educate and inform and I would like to think that no one wants to die prematurely, but if your only ambition in life is to suck down a pack a day or see the bottom of a bottle then perhaps talking to a someone who can give you an unbiased opinion about what's going on in your life could be the best medicine, not a cigarette or drinking your troubles away which is what we will look at next.

ALCOHOL

Just like smoking, alcohol also has obvious health risks and we won't go into too much detail but will cover some important things to keep in mind. Most of us love a drink or two... or three or four...and we all know that alcohol isn't the best for our health, aside from face planting the dash in your car because you thought a 40ft pine tree was your driveway, few people can tell you what the health risks of excessive alcohol consumption are. We all know that it affects the liver and that most people over 30 years old have fatty liver disease and don't even know it, furthermore, alcohol has been linked to more than 60 diseases including cancer. Alcohol can cause anaemia by depriving the red blood cells of oxygen, it can also cause cardiovascular disease by causing the platelets in your blood to clump together, in heavy drinkers alcohol can cause cirrhosis which is where the liver is so heavily scarred that it is no longer able to function. It can also cause the following:

Dementia, depression, gout, seizures, high blood pressure, infectious diseases, nerve damage, and pancreatitis in excessive drinkers, there is also a link to cancer of the breast, colon, liver and rectum.

Alcohol is another luxury that society has abused and due to its nature, it can just as easily take over your life like any illegal drug. Alcohol dependency or alcoholism is where you are dependent on alcohol to get you by, even if it's causing you physical harm or relationship problems with family and friends. People drink for so many reasons especially these days with the many stresses in our lives, work is a big one for most people especially when you're on a minimum wage or when your value isn't appreciated. Sometimes people drink to blow off steam after a tough week, or the occasional drinker may indulge at a wedding or a birthday but when the drink chooses the drinker due to chemical influence dictating over behavioural choice combined with a recent or ongoing cancer diagnosis then you have got a seriously tough battle ahead of you.

Alcohol that is linked to cancers of the upper digestive tract such as the mouth, oral pharynx, larynx, and oesophagus and is believed to carry a higher risk due to the synergism of smoking and drinking. In 2016 a study was conducted by Professor Jennie Connor at the Department of Preventive and Social Medicine, University of Otago, New Zealand called *"Alcohol consumption as a cause of cancer"* which concluded the following.

> *There is strong evidence that alcohol causes cancer at seven sites in the body and probably others. Current estimates suggest that alcohol-attributable cancers at these sites make up 5.8% of all cancer deaths worldwide. Confirmation of specific biological mechanisms by which alcohol increases the incidence of each type of cancer is not required to infer that alcohol is a cause.*

There are heaps of studies like this on the relationship between alcohol and cancer, so it goes without saying that if you have cancer already then you need to find a way to give it up. Now I'm not demonising alcohol, after all, you don't blame a gun for killing someone you blame the shooter right? Well in a sane world you do… I would be the biggest hypocrite going if I said I never drink or that we should ban alcohol or go back to the time of prohibition in the US. What I am saying is that we should be educating people on the long-term effects of alcohol consumption especially children, this way by the time they are

18 they can make informed decisions about whether they want to drink or not and not just let them buckle under social pressure which I'm sure everyone has had to deal with once or twice in their life particularly in their teen's. The ability of alcohol to hijack the brain and take over people lives is an all too familiar scene for some, personal tragedy can lead to excessive drinking and if you have been told you have cancer then you may be tempted to dull your senses with a bottle due to the perception that most people have about cancer and its treatment. The only solution to this is education, which is the key to understanding and listening to your body when it is telling you enough is enough.

Addictions cause problems which can be medical or psychological and there is always an expensive drug just waiting to fix it. When these problems are diagnosed by your doctor they will tell you to stop like it's an easy thing to do, they may even give you drugs to help cope with the stress of quitting. This is like giving a person who has a cold a tissue or a pain killer for their symptoms, it might help initially, but rarely are you told to stop eating shit and start living healthy, boost your immune system which would be addressing the underlying cause and not masking your symptoms.

My father had his battles with alcohol and when I was in my teens I just thought he liked to drink, it never occurred to me that he was running from something, from what I have no idea even to this day which is frustrating beyond measure because I will never know. They say that most people who are alcoholics are running from something and I guess the growing number of alcoholism and drug abuse in the world just goes to show that the world is not simple anymore and the pressure that's on people to achieve what society deems as normal is getting infinitely harder. I'm not anti-Australian when I say that the Aussie dream is dead and has been for a long time, the trouble is that the illusion of it remains which is why most people still think they have a shot at achieving it, and the US and many other countries are no different. Growing up my father and me never really talked about anything, we knew nothing about each other, he would say the same two things to me every day, good morning and good night and rarely anything in between, but when he had a drink then he would get chatty.

I guess the reason he drank as much as he did was to try and regain some kind of normality back into his life, or perhaps reflect on simpler and happier times, if my mother had allowed it I'm sure he would have drunk much more than he did. I'm not perfect either, far from it, while caring for my father I also abused alcohol and still do every now then. Back then I needed something to dull the monotony of having to tell people to stop what was obviously hurting them and everyone else around them, yet despite my warnings and predictions I was ignored. Even the debates with so-called experts which were stumped when I asked them the simplest of questions that they simply could not answer. Don't get the wrong idea, I was upset, frustrated, stressed, depressed and so angry I though id explode. I was also desperate to find a way to make my parent's see how ridiculous they were allowing my father to get a treatment that was failing him. As angry and hopeless as things felt I was never suicidal or anything like that, things would have gotten real simple for me if that's what I was thinking but where would that leave my family in their hour of need?

When I saw what everyone had to go through bearing my best friend's death I knew that I'd rather go down kicking and screaming like a spoilt brat than go out like that. Truthfully, I never understood people who wanted to kill themselves because they cannot handle what life throws at them, my logic has always been that if someone or something is causing me so much grief to make me want to kill myself then I would be more likely to kill the person causing my grief than killing myself. Think about it, why the fuck would you forfeit your existence when some asshole is the source of your anguish?

When it comes to life's challenges you do the best you can with what you've got, it's like what Matthew McConaughey said *"life isn't fair, never was, isn't now and never will be. Do not fall into the trap of entitlement, thinking that you are a victim, you are not"*. The point I'm getting at here is that if you have a dependency on alcohol then perhaps what is needed is for you to understand yourself better and discover why you are drinking so much or what your triggers are. Everyone is loved by someone and relationships no matter who they are with are always more important than drug or alcohol addiction, you should never be ashamed for seeking help for yourself no matter what it involves and if you have an alcohol addiction and you have cancer then instead of drinking yourself to death do something amazing with your life, you only get one. Try writing a book about your struggle, there are millions of people out there who can relate and who knows maybe by changing someone else's life you can change your own.

MEDICATIONS

More than 8 million people die every year from prescription medications given to them by their doctor, that's a death toll that far exceeds illegal drugs and even exceeds the death toll of the Vietnam War which started on November the 1st 1955 and finished on April 30th 1975. There are no questions, inquiries or anyone held accountable for why this murder by mistrust and flat out ignorance is allowed other than that's the way we have always done things.

We have been deceived into thinking that these deaths are a symptom of the disease or disorder that these people suffered from. Yet in many cases seemingly harmless drugs that are prescribed for pain relief, heartburn, cholesterol and many more turn out to be the catalyst for how these people died. Here are just some of the dozens of medications that had to be recalled due to them causing serious injury and even death.

- **Accutane (Isotretinoin)** –An acne cream which was found to be causing birth defects, miscarriages, premature births, bowel disease and suicidal tendencies, over 7,000 lawsuits were filed and was on the market for 27 years between 1982 to 2009.
- **Darvon & Darvocet (Propoxyphene)** – Was and Opioid pain reliever which caused serious toxicity to the heart and caused 2,110 deaths it was in the market for 55 years between 1955 and recalled in 2010.
- **Mylotarg (GemtuzumabOzogamicin)** – Was used for Acute Myeloid Leukaemia which caused an increased risk of death and veno-occlusive disease which is an obstruction of the veins. Was in use for 10 years between 2000 and 2010.

- **Rezulin (Troglitazone)** – An anti-diabetic and anti-inflammatory drug which caused at least 90 liver failures and 63 deaths, more than 35,000 claims were filed against Parker Davis/Werner Lambert now (Pfizer), was used for 3 years between 1997 and 2000.
- **Vioxx (Rofecoxib)** – (NSAID) used for pain relief which caused an increased risk of heart attack and stroke, was linked to more than 27,785 heart attacks or sudden cardiac deaths. Was in the market for 5 years between 1999 and 2004.

It's strange don't you think that a new drug which causes so much injury and death could be on the shelf practically overnight and stay there for years and even decades yet a promising anti-cancer drug has to undergo extensive clinical trials which could take 5 to 10 years and may not even pass.

As a rule of thumb if you ever get a prescription from your doctor ask them to print out a full list of side effects.

Then before you take the drug make a cup of tea sit at your computer and look them up, if they check out then you can at least say you were properly informed of the medication your doctor is prescribing, but if they are different do not be afraid to confront them considering you're the one who will have to live with whatever side effects you get. I guarantee that most doctors have no clue what is in half of these drugs they recommend and I'd bet that's because 99.9% of patients don't challenge them by checking, if they did doctors who blindly prescribe these medications would have a lot of explaining to do and lucky for them the law protects them so either way it makes no difference if they mess up.

There are some medications out there which have been implicated in causing or increasing your risk of certain cancers, for example, Hormone Replacement Therapy (HRT) which is used to treat women with menopause has been linked to an increased risk of breast cancer. Some other drugs commonly used for cholesterol, heartburn, blood pressure as well as creams used for eczema-like Elidel and Protopic may also cause cancer and why the FDA has officially warned people about the prolonged use of this product.

Without a doubt, we need to drastically change the way we view medications and come to terms with the fact that nature had all of this worked out at the beginning which is why most pharmaceutical grade drugs are synthesized from something in nature. Instead, companies have found a way to make a profit from drugs that appear to be harmless when in reality the side effects are so severe they should have never been approved for use in the first place.

Take Accutane for example, all these people wanted to do was get rid of a few pimples and now their children have birth defects and it was even shown to make people suicidal! That's a bit extreme just to get rid of some pimples don't you think? Don't get me wrong, there are people out there who cannot live without certain medications, but the greater question is, do we need them for everything? Most people wouldn't take a pain killer if a side effect was death and most people, like 99.9%, would agree that being dead was not the kind of pain relief they were looking for.

Medications can not only cause cancer but can make existing cancers worse by affecting the immune system. When it comes to medications, consider finding natural alternatives before resorting to more extreme measures, one that will simultaneously boost your immune system while attacking your condition directly. Going back to the dogma of medicine, there is a perception out there that natural treatments for conditions don't work because people do not see results right away. That is because unlike conventional medicine which hides symptoms, natural remedies are trying to heal your body by addressing the underlying cause which can take some time.

If you're a heavy user of medications which is defined as taking one or more pills daily then you should be speaking to your doctor about the side effects of stopping these drugs and seeking other opinions about safer alternatives. You won't know until you ask the question, and you may be surprised by the answer.

THOUGHTS, FEELINGS & EMOTIONS

A person's thoughts, feelings and emotional state should not be underestimated! This aspect of the human body is completely disregarded in conventional medicine as they only focus on the physical/mechanical aspects of the human body. But science also confirms that the body is nothing but energy, and your thoughts, feelings and emotions can affect this energy.

There are no strong studies that show stress can cause cancer but there are studies that show what stress does to the body and let's face it, in this day and age who isn't stressed? I was stressed writing this book, but that kind of stress is not the kind of stress I'm talking about. I am referring to the stress caused by major life events such as the death of a loved one, losing your job, your home, a divorce, child custody battles, financial stress, or perhaps you are experiencing emotional stress because your partner cheated on you, these are the kinds of stress events that can change everything.

Today it is estimated that 9 out of 10 visits to the doctor are stress-related and it probably doesn't help when you have to wait more than an hour just to see one. If you ask a person with cancer what was going on in their life around the time they got diagnosed many of them will say that they were under huge amounts of stress, that's because mental and emotional stress can create physiological changes in the body.

Science has shown that chronic long-term stress can lead to hormone imbalances, digestive problems, fertility problems, urinary problems and even weaken the immune system, stress can be either physical, mental or emotional and sometimes a combination of all depending on what has happened. When people are under stress, they tend to lean on unhealthy habits to get them through intense down periods such as drinking, smoking and even binge eating. Though alcohol can be used as a temporary fix for the problem it can easily lead to addiction in these people and won't address the root cause of the problem, smoking is just flat out bad for you there are no positives to it and binge eating isn't good for you either because you will probably eat all the things you shouldn't like take away foods and things that are high in sugar and saturated fats making your condition worse.

In a study called *"Psychological stress and the risk of breast cancer: a case-control study"* by the Institute of Physical Education, Faculty of Natural Sciences, University of Szczecin, Al. Piastów Szczecin, Poland they concluded the following.

After adjustment for age and other potential confounders, we found that women with major life events, the stress of daily activity, and depression had 3.7 times higher risk for breast cancer, compared to those which did not experience such stress.

Whatever is going on in your life you must realise that the way you think and feel about it has to change because nothing stays the same forever. For example, when someone suffers a trauma or life event that causes physical, mental or emotional harm, it may leave its mark on this person for many years leaving them angry, frustrated, depressed, violent and even suicidal. Some of these emotions were probably necessary at the time for you to cope. Take anger for example, at the time your anger may have been useful to you coping with what was happening but now that time has passed you are no longer in the same place, so your anger is no longer serving you, instead, this anger you feel has now turned in to self-sabotage stopping you from moving on and making your peace with what has happened. I personally felt this way after everything that had happened so I know there is some truth to this statement.

The things that happened in my family over the years should never have happened, we all have our demons and at the time I did not realize that my parents and my sister were battling their own, in the end, I was reduced to a spectator as everything I had predicted happened right in front of me and there was absolutely nothing I could say or do to change their minds. If the source of your anguish lies with other people and you are trying to talk reason to a highly emotional person you will raise a wall that will never be lowered and every time you talk about these particular issues you will get an argument. Every time I would tell my mother and father about the things I learned about cancer they never took me seriously because what I was telling them was so detached from what they knew that they just couldn't believe that any of it could be true.

The reason I am even sharing this is that my situation is not unique, there are people out there who have endured far worse than me and my family, but I know that when it comes to your attitude I would rather be happy doing my own thing than miserable just to please others. People always view negative experiences as this emotional wall that cannot be climbed, but in truth, we learn our most valuable lessons from failure, not our success. If you always got things right then you would never learn anything and how boring and mundane would that be?

People have a way of making you doubt and question yourself in just about everything, these people will hinder your progress in life because the truth is they are going nowhere and they know it!

If you do a bit of research on cancer survivors who have used natural treatments many of them will say that having cancer was the best thing that happened to them, it scared them so much that it forced them to change their lifestyle and make them focus on what it means to be happy. Many of these people say that they are now living richer and fuller lives than they did before and are happier now than they have ever been because they are not succumbing to the impossible standards that society demands of us. Happiness is relative, it could be 1 million dollars in the bank for one person or downgrading the home to a small shack in the country and living off the land to another. Happiness and stress are opposites, you wouldn't be stressed if you were happy about your life, you are stressed because you are not happy about your life and things are not going your way. To truly achieve happiness, you have to ask yourself what does happiness mean to you?

I have always said that a simple life is a good life, you don't need to complicate it with materialism which has been drilled into our heads to keep us focussed on this consumer-driven society.

Whatever the underlying issues are you need to realise that happiness is a place that is achieveable to everyone, you just have to redefine it for yourself. Maybe having cancer is the wake-up call you needed to change your life and not the death sentence your doctor tells you. Not I or anyone else can fix your problems, talking to someone about your problems is an intellectual process to get you to understand what it is you need to do, but there will come a point where the action needed must come from you, you cannot envoke real change through thought alone. To do this you need to find ways to de-stress, this could be burning incense, getting a massage, spend a day at the beach, go on a camping trip, play peaceful music, take that extra nap or download a guided meditation video to help you sleep and relax. If you hate your job don't go, you have cancer for God sake! Tell your boss they can shove their job up their ass. Whatever your poison is for relaxing and destressing do it, it's like what Gandhi said, a man is but a product of his thoughts, what he thinks he becomes.

PART IV

CHAPTER 12: CONSPIRACY OR CRIME?

In February 2013 my father completed another round of chemo and radiation and was told he was in the clear, again he interpreted this to mean that I was wrong and that the doctors were right, despite their premature assessment. The doctors had told my family that medically he is fine, but my mother and sister did not think this at all. My mother described him at times as a completely different person and there had been several occasions where he would look at my mother and sister with absolute disgust. They described it to me as a glare of intense hatred and disgust making them feel worthless, then again if you got radiation on your fucking brain who knows how bad your eggs get scrambled? Doctors, especially oncologists are trained to give you what you respond to, not what heals you, there is a world of difference. After 12 months my father's vagueness had persisted which we had all put down to the radiation and I began to let my guard down thinking that the worse of it was behind us.

In February 2014 on another routine check-up, we had learned that his cancer had recurred and the oncologist was recommending the same chemo drug that didn't work the last time. Unfortunately, this is the mentality of most oncologists, I would have preferred he take no drugs and do what is suggested in this book, even if I was to subject my father to the madness of conventional treatment why would I use a drug that didn't work before? As far as conspiracies go the "Cancer Conspiracy" which is not a conspiracy at all, it's a crime, and is among the worst and the most deceiving. It plays on the trust people have for their doctor and assumes that they are always adequately informed on the drugs and treatments they prescribe to their patients.

The conditioning for this false belief goes back to primary school, don't believe me? Then ask a child, where do you go when you are sick? They will say either the doctor or the hospital, and who works at the hospital? Even a child knows this, so why do adults struggle to understand that when you go to the doctor for an illness it's because that's what you have been conditioned to do!

So before we get carried away let's define the word conspiracy and put it into context so you can understand exactly what is being said to you. In society today just uttering that word instils a level of disbelief that makes it almost impossible for you to talk to people about certain issues. These kinds of people are full of opinions that mean absolutely nothing because they are not valid opinions, opinions based on nothing are worthless because they are only looking at a problem from one perspective. Society has created an alternative meaning to the word conspiracy and this is largely to do with the way the media have used it. According to the Oxford dictionary, a conspiracy is defined as *"a secret plan by a group to do something unlawful or harmful"*. So if this is the definition of a conspiracy then conspiracies are going on all of the fucking time! Was it a conspiracy when Johnson & Johnson lied about the asbestos in their talcum powder for 40 years? Or when Monsanto's lied about their herbicide Round-Up-Ready being safe to use and was biodegradable to the environment? Or that a baby's immune system can handle as many as 10,000 vaccinations?

Every single day these things are going on and people have no clue because they don't understand the definition or the context in which they are used. So why is there so much resistance and lack of acceptance by people when the media does this?

The answer is simple, the public is suffering from a belief in something and are not making logical choices based on facts.

Another example is the word UFO, I have personally witnessed three UFO's in my lifetime, if I was too openly tell people what I saw society would not treat me kindly and that's because people have no idea what I just said to them. I said I saw a UFO meaning an "Unidentified Flying Object," I never said that I saw aliens although that is a possibility, I saw lights in the sky which did not behave or resemble any aircraft that I know of, so by definition alone the account is a UFO. People's understanding of the word "Conspiracy" is the same as that of a UFO, they think what the media wants them to not what the account really is.

So to find the truth we must not confuse the facts with our beliefs, and also our many bias's which make up what we perceive reality to be, we must learn to look at these problems objectively and view them with a logical and rational mind. Many people cannot distinguish the difference between fact and belief, this because some peoples beliefs are facts to them and this is how they identify with the world. This is what happens when people use their emotional brain instead of their logical brain when making decisions about what to believe.

Over the years I have found many religious people to fall into this category especially on the subject of God, we do not know for a fact if God exists and just because people believe in one doesn't make it true. I'm not saying there isn't a God, only that peoples minds should be open to the possibility that if there is a God it may not be what we expect.

Before we begin the next chapter I want to also define a fact and a belief so there is no ambiguity about what is being said, my research over the years has taught me to see this subject as a crime against humanity not a conspiracy by definition.

Fact: A thing that is known or proved to be true

Belief: 1. An acceptance that something exists or is true, especially one without proof.

2. Trust, faith, or confidence in (someone or something)

I have always been an advocate of asking questions especially if they are tough or make people feel uncomfortable, how else will we learn if we are always comfortable in our surroundings? Jason Bacchetta said it best *"I don't feel threatened by people who ask questions. It's those who refuse to answer them that frightens me".*

Now things have been put into context let's take a look at some brave and amazing people who tried to bring us a treatment for cancer in the last 100 years and how corporations and the authorities shut them down so you would be forced to buy their toxic drugs instead.

Conspiracy or Crime?

Conspiracy theories are things people often make fun of until they are right, then everyone else looks stupid for not seeing what was going on. People also say the same thing about preppers, they make fun of them calling them paranoid, but when shit goes down they are the other "P word" PREPARED, again everyone else is left to suffer because they refuse to believe the facts in front of them.

So far we have looked at quite a few controversial issues and without a doubt, these are genuine crimes, not conspiracy theories. It is not theoretical what is happening on these issues because both sides recognise that it's being done, the difference is half of them BELIEVE these things to be good whereas the FACTS demonstrate they are not. Critics on issues like the ones raised in this book in my opinion often fall into one of these 3 categories:

1. They either know about the problem because they are a part of it, and are deliberately misleading the masses.
2. They have been lied to by those responsible by fabricating science to gain their persuasive power and influence.
3. Finally, they are just willfully ignorant about the problem because it does not fit into their model of reality.

It would also be very biased of me if I said that all critics were wrong which is simply not the case, the problem with a book like this one is that there is an abundance of evidence that contradicts the mainstream narrative but who is going to read it all? Simply ignoring facts is not a persuasive argument by any standard, yet that appears to be the mainstream position.

Nutrition Could Kill You

These days nutrition will kill you and I don't mean that eating organic fruit and vegetables are going to have you pushing up daisies, what I mean is that if you are a practising nutritionist or holistic doctor and are an advocate for natural/alternative medicine then you could be up shit creek with no paddle.

It's no secret that Big Pharma's number one enemy is alternative medicine and that more and more people thanks to the internet are waking up and realising that there does exist more options than surgery, chemotherapy and radiation for the typical cancer patient. In fact, according to Dr Leonard Coldwell one of the world's leading self-help experts on beating cancer, there are more than 400 cancer treatments that cost next to nothing and are side effect free. Dr Leonard Coldwell also successfully treated his mother with Hepatitis C, Liver cirrhosis and liver cancer in the terminal state with the prognosis of 6 months to live over 40 years ago and today raises awareness and educates people on what they can do to help beat their cancer without conventional treatment. He is also the author of 19 bestselling books and thousands of publications and hundreds of CD and DVD self-help systems, so if you have cancer he is the doctor for you, his website also claims a 92.3% Success rate. You can visit it at www.drleonardcoldwellbio.com

In the last 5 years, the mainstream media has kept the killing of holistic doctors in the United States to themselves and refuse to acknowledge that any of them are connected. According to Erin Elizabeth who is a huge activist for the healing arts and founder of website Health Nut News which is in the top 20 most viewed health websites in the world, more than 100 holistic doctors and naturopaths have died in the most bizarre circumstances. From murder to suicides and dissapearances never to be seen again, drugs, stabbings, hit and runs, car crashes and shootings you name it, it has all happened to these people and most of the US had no idea. Law enforcement had only recently recognised that perhaps these strange circumstances are connected and has only now started to consult the FBI. 100 deaths in 3 years let alone in mysterious circumstances would convince any court in the world that something is going on. They say that 3 coincidences are a conspiracy right? Well, what the hell do you call 100? Scarier still is that as I was writing this book I had to keep coming back to this chapter to change the figure because more and more people just kept dying. When I first caught wind of the death toll it was around 10 or 12 which at the time I thought was mind-blowing and that was early 2017.

The first death started on June 19th, 2015 Father's Day, Dr Jeffery Bradstreet who was big on alternative medicine and had dedicated his career to intensive Autism research which helped many children using a therapy called Globulin Component Macrophage Activity Factor or GcMAF. GcMAF is a type of immunotherapy; it is an essential protein that our body produces which has 6 attacks on cancer and 20 beneficial attacks on disease. Without GcMAF the immune system collapses and the disease or cancer can become chronic to acute, if applied externally the attack resumes within minutes and stage 4 cancer patients improved within the first week, there is also a 25% reduction in tumour size and within 6 months a cancer patient could be as cancer-free as anyone else.

Dr Bradstreet had dedicated his career to Autism due to a family incident where and he had approved the use of a vaccine as many parents do. It was highly suspected of causing his sons Autism and after this incident, he felt compelled to right this wrong by helping children with the disorder. During his time among the living, he helped more than 2000 Autistic children using GcMAF, where 15% of patients had no changes, 85% improved to some degree and where 15% of the 85% had their Autism eradicated. The Huffington Post and other media had labelled him an anti-vaccine quack, which according to his family said that he admitted that vaccines have had harmful effects on children's immune systems and that in some instances had even killed them, but he never said he was anti-vaccine. His family believe that they just wanted to discredit him even though none of them claiming he was an anti-vaccine quack had read any of his research.

Naturally, this was just the beginning, over the next 6 months chiropractors, osteopaths and holistic doctors were going missing or turning up dead until late December 2015 when the focus shifted to cancer researchers. One cancer researcher Professor Alan Clarke at age 52 was found dead hanging from a tree in woodlands wearing a rubber suit, the authorities ruled his death as accidental, which is just ridiculous! How the fuck do you accidentally hang yourself? And why would you be in a rubber suit in the woods to do it? Either he planned to kill himself or it was a murder staged as a suicide. Yet this incident was not an isolated event and the bloodshed continued. On June the 16th 2016 a man walked into the office of another holistic doctor and shot him, turned the gun on himself for a murder-suicide.

The day after on the 17th of June 2016 a man walked into the office of Dr Tiejun Huang PhD/MD with a knife a killed him in cold blood. Another death was on the 11th of January 2018 when a 67-year-old doctor called Clive Bridgham was murdered in his home, this was covered by the news and even the police describe it as a targeted attack and was not random.

Erin Elizabeth has documented these findings and she was even friends with some of these doctors so for more information on the circumstances surrounding these peoples deaths please go to www.healthnutnews.com. Erin Elizabeth has also mentioned certain death threats for getting the information into the public domain. I guess if there was nothing to it she wouldn't be getting threatened which only adds more weight to the argument that there is something to cover up and a plot of some kind in the works.

Those who think this is fantasy or the product of an overactive imagination try telling that to the autistic people that were helped by GcMAF or the families of those who have been murdered. Ask yourself why to date that not one oncologist or radiologist has been killed in the same manner? Treatments like GcMAF could have revolutionised the way we treat many disease's and not just cancer. Maybe these people were killed because they were too honest and outspoken on these controversial issues like Dr Teresa Sievers who was very outspoken about vaccine safety. Each one of these people has a story to tell and at face value, it appears like the competition is being killed off, but that is just my opinion. Erin also said that Dr John Marshall, another victim, was a 4th generation marine with 2 tours of Afganistan and survival training, plus he worked out all the time, he then goes for a jog one day along a river, slips in and drowns... Really? And people are expected to believe this shit?

The police have now concluded that it may have been a homicide and they have decided to reopen the case.

In September 2015 a similar incident happened in Germany at a naturopathic conference in Handel oh where 29 holistic doctors and naturopaths were poisoned with a toxic dose of amphetamine. Fortunately, none died, but many were close to death as ambulances and 150 personnel rushed to help them. The first respondents said it was a horrific scene as the victims were in the front yard of the conference in agonising pain suffering from delusions, breathing problems, heart and cramp conditions and some in life-threatening situations. An investigation was immediately done and it was concluded that the consumption of the toxic dose of amphetamine was not self-inflicted and that it may have been a deliberate and malicious act. Investigations are still pending and as of yet, no one has been held accountable for this attack on natural medicine. Despite the lack of evidence it appears to be deliberate attack on natural medicine like the string of murders and suicides in the US. It's also reasonable to assume that those responsible are the ones who stand to profit the most from their deaths, as the simplest explanation is often the correct one. Logic 101 dictates that this is a message to anyone wanting to practice this dying art. No doubt there will be some sceptic that says it could have just been a crazy person in a random attack, which is stupid because obviously, this person is crazy, the real question I want answered is did they do it alone or were they under instruction from someone else? To the best of my knowledge this person/persons is still out there and they may even be connected to the string of murders in the US, but one thing is for certain, I have yet to see an attack like this on any oncologist or radiologist considering what they are told to put people through in the name of treatment.

You may be thinking these events are unfortunate but they don't constitute a conspiracy, well not on their own they don't, but when you look into the past you realise that this is nothing more than history repeating itself where the American Medical Association (AMA) refused to acknowledge the medical pioneers in our past bringing positive results to patients and were punished for doing so simply because they held no medical licence.

Over the last century, many people have tried to come out with their breakthrough treatments for cancer and other diseases that were natural and cost next to nothing. For years this information has been trying to come out and the mainstream medical community refuses to acknowledge it despite people all over the world healing themselves without medical intervention. The pioneers for this new age thinking were harassed, arrested and even threatened with death because of the hope they represented and the profits they threatened. This is why today most doctors don't even know who they are or anything about their research. This suppression goes back to the 1920s and is how long they have been sitting on a viable treatment for cancer with no harmful side effects, the woman responsible for this was Renee Cassie.

Rene Caisse

In the mid-1920s Rene M. Caisse was the head nurse at the Sisters of Providence Hospital in a northern Ontario town. One day she had observed an elderly patient with a scar on her breast and asked her about it, she told Rene that she had breast cancer 30 years ago when she migrated from England to Ontario. She said that her right breast became sore, swollen and very painful and that her husband had taken her to Toronto where doctors had told her that she had advanced breast cancer and that it needed to be removed fast or she would die. During a prospecting trip with her husband, she was approached by an old Indian medicine man who told her the same thing except he knew how to treat it, being broke they could not afford the surgery and she did not want her breast removed, so her and her husband went with the medicine man where he showed them certain herbs in the fields and said to make a tea out of them and to drink it every single day until its gone. The woman was 80 years old when she told Rene this story and so Rene wrote down the ingredients to the tea that treated her patient's breast cancer.

A few months later Rene's aunt, her mother's sister, had developed stomach cancer with liver involvement and was given 6 months to live by her doctor. Rene met Dr R.O Fisher of Toronto her auntie's physician and asked if he would supervise the herbal treatment that was given to her by her patient, as conventional medicine could no longer help, Dr Fisher didn't see the harm in trying and so he agreed. In short, the herbal concoction had successfully treated her auntie's cancer and she lived a bright and long 21 years after modern medicine had told her she was going to die, the treatment also had no side effects and her aunty had no reoccurrences after that time.

On October 27th, 1926 eight doctors who had witnessed the amazing effects of Rene's herbal tea on cancer agreed to sign a petition to the Department of National Health and Welfare at Ottawa which asked that Rene be given the appropriate facilities to develop the treatment further and continue her research. The petition read:

To Whom It May Concern:

We the undersigned believe that the "Treatment for Cancer" given by Nurse R.M. Caisse can do no harm and that it relieves pain, will reduce the enlargement and will prolong life in hopeless cases.

To the best of our knowledge, she has not been given a case to treat until everything in medical and surgical science has been tried without effect and even then she was able to show remarkable beneficial results on those cases at that late stage.

We would be interested to see her given an opportunity to prove her work in a large way. To the best of our knowledge, she has treated all cases free of any charge and has been carrying on this work over the period of the past two years.

The Department of National Health responded to this letter by sending two of their doctors, only to have her arrested for practicing medicine without a medical licence even though her actions were overseen by a licenced doctor. However, this was only the beginning, during her lifetime Renee had endured nearly 50 years of persecution from authority figures, government and those in the medical profession all for actually healing people's cancer. In their eyes the results didn't matter and their only argument was that she was not an officially trained or a licenced doctor.

The trouble Rene had then is the same trouble we have today, if you can heal a persons cancer but science cannot explain how then it's quackery or pseudoscience. I love science but its not the most humble profession, mainstream science likes to think that it always has an answer, just like a politician who is full of shit! Instead, their answer to this problem is to lock you up saying you don't have a licence even though the ingredients were natural, legal and without any side effects, this is nothing more than a way for them to control who gives advice on disease and who can legally give treatment. The problem is then compounded when these herbs are successful in treating disease because they are cheap and easy to grow, unlike the production of expensive drugs which is a direct threat to the establishment's profits. Legally, biotech companies cannot patent something that exists naturally, it has to be genetically modified before they claim it under intellectual property law and this is a huge reason why organic plants like marijuana and even apricot seeds which have been proven to have a positive effect on cancer cells are banned in countries like the US as a treatment for cancer.

Renee eventually gave up working as a nurse and spent her time working out of the basement in her mother's house where she had made her lab to do more research. Doctors would often send patients to her apartment when they knew they could no longer help them and it got to the point where she was treating as many as 30 people a day. She decided to call her herbal tea

ESSIAC which was her last name spelt backwards, she said it herself that she had lost count of how many times she was threatened with arrest and imprisonment for treating people with ESSIAC without a medical licence, but she knew there were no side effects so in her eyes there was nothing to fear.

Rene had finally got approval to open the Rene Caisse Cancer Clinic, where she was treating between 300-600 people a week and did so for roughly 8 years, however, the AMA and FDA would still not approve ESSIAC to be legalised. After a special visit by Dr Leonardo from Buffalo he said to Rene *"so you think you have a cure for cancer?"*

She laughed and said that she doesn't think, she knows, and agreed to let the doctor check Rene's patients to see the results for himself, to which he said, *"it looks like you have a cure for cancer, but the medical establishment will never let you get away with it"*.

For years Rene had refused to give the exact formula to labs and universities because she knew if she did it would get buried and that would be the end of it, however, a mysterious group of entrepreneur's approached her and offered Rene 1 million dollars for the exact formula, but she refused because they would not guarantee that the formula would be made free to anyone who needed it. On a side note, I know that you don't offer someone 1 million dollars even by today's standards if you think what they have is worthless or doesn't work.

Rene continued to try and legalise her ESSIAC treatment and even got a petition signed with 55,000 signatures including many patients and doctors, but after going before the legislator to have it approved she had lost by 3 votes! I mean C'mon seriously... 3 votes and there's no crime or conspiracy on cancer...

Soon after Rene's clinic was closed down where she had a nervous breakdown, she could not handle sick patients dying of cancer and begging her to treat them when she had been told by the authorities and medical establishment to stop. Later in 1958, Rene was asked to have ESSIAC tested by a clinic in Massachusetts, by director Charles Brush MD who was the personal physician to President John F Kennedy and he concluded that ESSIAC was non-toxic and that it did have an effect on cancer. But even after this the FDA still outlawed and forbid the use of ESSIAC as a cancer treatment, they came up with a whole bunch of bullshit excuses which made no sense at all, this then escalated into patients suing the FDA for denying the public a cure for cancer, which is exactly what we should be doing today!

This is but a simplified version of the events in Rene's story and it is a real eye-opener, just thinking that alternative cancer treatment has been around since the 1920s shows the level of manipulation and control these corporations have over our government and why we will never get the fruits of their labour if we ask for it.

For more information on Rene Caisse and her tea ESSIAC go to. www.essiacinfo.org

I decided to concentrate on Rene Caisse's work as opposed to the many others in our history who tried to make their treatments mainstream knowledge for a couple of reasons. The first is that it illustrates perfectly how long the medical profession has been sitting on a real cancer treatment and the other is her use of natural herbs, that were fairly common in Native America and easy to get today.

The truth is that there are so many people that have tried to bring this kind of information to light and have been aggressively pursued to the point of fines, arrests, courts, jail and even death threats all because they have challenged the status quo, and of all of them that could have fought back none did it better than Harry Hoxsey.

Harry Hoxsey

Harry Hoxsey was a successful entrepreneur in the oil business and had repeated lawsuits against the AMA and eventually the FDA of which some he won. His cancer treatment is said to have come from his grandfather, a veterinarian who in the 1840s observed a horse recover from cancer by eating certain weeds in a field which Harry then applied to treating cancer in people. The Hoxsey clinic is said to have an 80% or higher recovery for cancer patients including those who have been abandoned by orthodox oncology.

Harry Hoxsey began to rock the apple cart with his claims of healing cancer in his book called “You don’t need to die”. When the AMA caught wind of Hoxsey’s claims they sent author and journalist James Wakefield Burke to essentially debunk Hoxsey’s cancer cure claims and label him the quack they thought he was. James Wakefield only intended to stay the day which turned into 6 weeks where he became fascinated by the results Hoxsey’s clinic produced.

He then wrote an article called the "The quack that cured cancer" but the press refused to release it not wanting to add fuel to a situation they couldn't control. As far as disbelievers go there was no one more set on getting rid of Hoxsey than district attorney Al Templeton who had arrested Hoxsey more than 100 times in 2 years. Hoxsey was also known to carry $10,000 in cash so he could make bail, that's how ridiculous it got! According to James Wakefield Burke sometimes Harry would deliberately stay in jail so all the people he had helped would come and bring food, sing and pray, embarrassing the authorities for arresting him in the first place. After appearing in court many times none of Hoxsey's patients would testify against him because he had saved their life where conventional doctors had failed. It wasn't until Al Templeton's brother Mike got terminal cancer did he secretly go to Hoxsey to treat his brother's cancer and when he did he gave Hoxsey the credit and became an advocator to Hoxsey's cause.

At one point there were as many as 17 Hoxsey clinics all over the US which were shut down by the FDA and it wasn't because they didn't successfully treat cancer, they were shut down because his clinics were not approved by the FDA which if you haven't learned by now was never going to happen. However, there remains one clinic which was founded in 1963 in Tijuana, Baja California Mexico called the Hoxsey Bio-Medical Centre, if you want to learn more or get a consultation I suggest going to their website www.hoxseybiomedical.com.

There is also a documentary you can YouTube which is quite old but attests to how long this has all been known, it's called Hoxsey when healing becomes a crime by Ken Ausubel and

Catherine Salveson. Despite Hoxsey's fame and power, he was still no match for the authorities proving that they will let nothing threaten their empire which has been built on the back of people's suffering. However, another man who found a successful treatment for cancer by trying to alleviate his medical condition was none other than Max Gerson.

Max Gerson

Max Gerson was born in Wongrowitz, Germany in 1881, the story of Max Gerson and how he created the Gerson therapy arose from a great need to rid himself of terrible migraines which he had believed was to do with his diet. It was a painstaking process of trial and error, eating nothing but apples he would add or remove certain foods that would trigger a migraine and this was how the Gerson Therapy was born. He then started to treat his patients with the migraine treatment until one day a patient of his said that his diet had also healed their skin Tuberculosis. Max had also gained a famous friend during this time, a man by the name of Albert Schweitzer, M.D who just happened to be a Nobel Peace Prize winner and a talented theologian, musician, philosopher and physician. Max had also completely healed Albert Schweitzer's wife of lung tuberculosis, and until the end of his life in 1958, they remained close friends. Max's treatment was also able to completely rid 446 out of 450 skin tuberculosis in a carefully monitored clinical trial.

In 1958 after 30 years of clinical experimentation, Gerson published his book called "A Cancer Therapy: Results of 50 cases". When Max Died in 1959 Albert Schweitzer gave the following eulogy.

"...I see in him one of the most eminent geniuses in the history of medicine. Many of his basic ideas have been adopted without having his name connected with them. Yet, he has achieved more than seemed possible under adverse conditions. He leaves a legacy which commands attention and which will assure him his due place. Those whom he has cured will now attest to the truth of his ideas."

Today there are two Gerson clinics one in Tijuana Mexico and the other in Hungary Europe, if you want to learn more about the Gerson therapy then visit the website at www.gerson.org or read one of the many books they have on offer for treating cancer and chronic diseases in a non-toxic way.

These are just some of the people in our history that we do not hear about today because the mainstream medical community labels them as quack's playing doctor even though the results speak for themselves. These are the people who were shunned for challenging the status quo and they did it for you!

Despite persecution and adversity, these people dedicated their lives to bringing this knowledge to the public domain so we could be disease and cancer-free and the powers that be said no! Below are a few more people worth mentioning as some of them have also endured persecution from the authorities for their work despite their promising results.

- **Dr Leonard Coldwell** – Known for his alternative cancer diet and author of "The Only Answer to Cancer" and many more self-help systems. www.drleonardcoldwellbio.com
- **Dr Stanislaw R. Burzynski** – For his research on Antineoplastons, www.burzynskiclinic.com

- **Dr Tullio Simoncini** – Bicarbonate and the fungus theory of cancer, not genetics www.curenaturalicancro.com
- **Jason Vale** – Who was imprisoned for selling Apricot Kernels after he treated his own cancer with them. www.apricotsfromgod.info
- **Chris Beat Cancer** - Youtube Channel - Has more than 120,000 subscribers and has even appeared on The Ricki Lake show telling people how he beat his cancer on a raw food diet.

It should be obvious by now based on these people's experiences that something is not quite right and there is more we could be doing to explore these revolutionary treatments. It would appear that there is an attempt to block progress in the current medical establishment and if a cancer cure is found then it is to be controlled or contained in a way that doesn't interfere with the billions of dollars of profit that Big Pharma makes on the current system.

Over the years there has been an attempt to get people off the land by making them dependant on a system that is designed to trap and enslave them with no concern for their wellbeing and governments have facilitated this process. This is exactly how slavery starts and those too naive to see it for what it is are incapable of connecting the dots and seeing that cancer causation, treatment, information control and suppression are just one part of a grand lie that we have all been living. We are at a stage in our history where we don't need the government to do anything because we have become so accustomed to our complacency that we are self-regulating our slavery, and all the government needs to do is deal with the few that disagree.

For a while now researchers like Jim Marrs in his book called "Population Control – How Corporate Owners Are Killing us" have been talking about a plan to kill as many as 90-95% of the world's population. This agenda is for the elite like Bill Gates and the Clintons to control people and how fast the Earths finite resources are being used. There is also evidence that an elite group working within a shadow government has adopted a philosophy akin to that of the Georgia guides stones which were mysteriously erected in 1980. In 12 different languages including ancient Sumerian, the Georgia guide stones describe how to rebuild humanity after a catastrophic event, the very first rule says to keep the population under 500 million people. With the current population at 7.9 billion and set to explode to 9.6 billion by the year 2050, this may not be a stretch of the imagination, especially now we have COVID 19 and big pharma's vaccine which will soon be mandatory for everyone sooner or later.

Here is the Georgia Guide Stones.

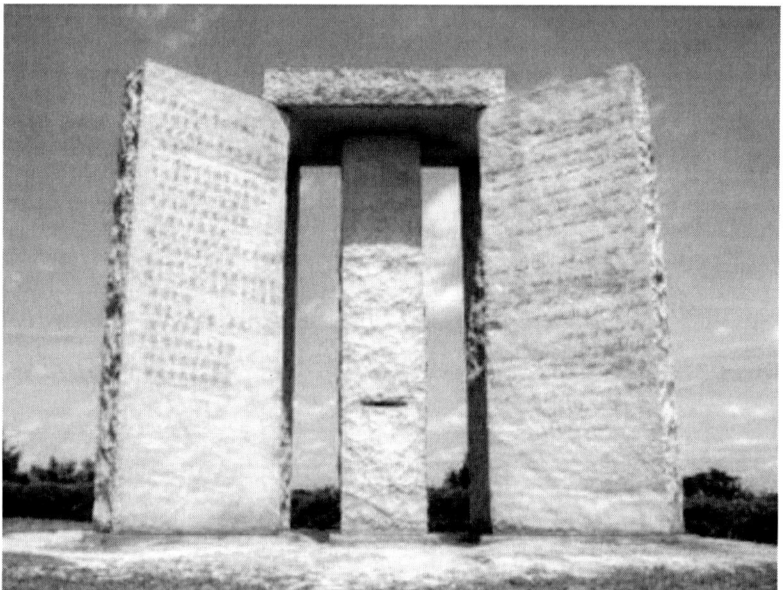

When it comes to the uncertainty of our future I often think about the movie Elysium with Matt Damon and wonder if that's what our future looks like. In some ways its already happening with the elite living in luxury looking down on the rest of us as they often do, disgusted at even breathing the same air. I think about this and human nature and think perhaps it's not so far-fetched, of course, this is just one of the things I think about when I see and hear all of the crazy shit going on in our world today.

When you see and hear all of the wars, famine, disease, poverty and cancer slowly becoming the number one killer in the world, it makes sense that this is how you would go about killing 95% of the population, because if it were done openly to us there is no way we would stand for it.

If you think that this is the product of an overactive imagination then perhaps you should google some of the multi-million dollar bunkers the elite are building from ex nuclear missile silos for themselves all over the world, they are scared and I reckon they know something is coming. Why would the wealthy and powerful build them if there was nothing to worry about in our future? It's so catastrophically logical when you look at it from that perspective, but don't take my word for it just turn on the TV and watch the news every night and you'll catch on.

People may say it's a bold statement to label corporations as terrorists, but the definition of terrorism is *"A person who uses unlawful violence and intimidation, especially against civilians, in the pursuit of political aims"* which has been a reoccurring theme throughout this book. In fact, by comparison, the threat of foreign terrorists and Islamic extremists and the casualties inflicted by them are minuscule at best in comparison to corporations. To put it into perspective the Napoleon wars killed between 3.5 and 6 million people, the Vietnam wars killed between 800,000 and 3.5 million people, WWI killed approximately 40 million people and WWII killed approximately 56 million people just in military and civilians, not including the disease and famine in the aftermath. Yet if cancer is killing more than 8 million people each year and growing fast, then in less than 8 years cancer would have killed more people than any of these wars, so why isn't it getting the attention it deserves? That means that 1 in every 6 deaths in the world today is a cancer death and in terms of frequency, Australia is number 3 in the world which is no surprise because most Australians are away with the fucking fairies.

Look at how much rubbish we are sold on the war on terrorism because of the unspeakable deaths that have come from it, yet prescription drugs for cancer treatment have a death toll that completely dwarfs terrorism and yet not a single thing is mentioned about it. So ask yourself, by definition does a genuine conspiracy exist? And how long will we tolerate these crimes against humanity?

CHAPTER 13: CUT, POISON, BURN

This is where we take a look at the conventional treatment of cancer and why it has a high probability of failure. We will be looking at surgery, chemotherapy, radiation therapy and also gene therapy and why in most cases it will accelerate your cancer and could ultimately lead to your death. Statistically, you are only cancer-free unless you survive beyond the 5-year threshold from your original diagnosis. This means that if you died 5 years and 1 day after you have been diagnosed you are statistically a cancer survivor even though you are dead, just another clever way for them to sell the lie that conventional treatment works.

Surgery, Chemo, and radiation have been around for a long time, surgery as a means to treat cancer goes back nearly 200 years and radiation as early as the 1890s. Chemo was discovered in the 1940s and yet even though the techniques and technologies have changed the prevailing philosophy and approach to treating cancer has not.

SURGERY

Surgery is by far the safest conventional treatment for cancer. Skin cancer or melanomas are often surgically removed and are rarely fatal in comparison to other types of cancer. Remember, cancer is a systemic metabolic disease from a dysfunctional metabolism, not something that can be fixed long term with a scalpel.

It is also common for people to get chemo after surgery and there are two reasons for this, your cancer may have small colonies of cells floating around your bloodstream just waiting to settle and metastasize which they use chemotherapy to target these colonies.

The other is a bit more sinister, a biopsy used to diagnose your type of cancer could easily do the same thing. This is called "Seeding" and occurs when cancerous tissue has contaminated health tissue by diagnostic or surgical procedures given to you by your doctor. So ask yourself, what are the odds that your doctors could remove your cancer surgically without contaminating healthy tissue? This is why chemotherapy is given after surgery and is standard practice!

There is a growing number of scientific evidence that points to surgery-induced metastasis and in the vast majority of cases, metastasis is what kills the patient, not the primary tumour. Breakaway cells from the primary tumour that enter the bloodstream are picked up by your immune system and are usually killed posing no threat, however, for cancer to metastasize it has to go through quite a few obstacles before this can be achieved. A cancer cell has to first make its way through the connective tissue surrounding the primary tumour which is like a membrane containing all the cancer cells. It will then try to get access to the lymph system or your bloodstream, it does this by secreting enzymes which breaks down the tissue walls and landing on a blood vessel, it secretes more enzymes and tries to hitch a ride into the bloodstream which is like the bodies freeway. This is where the immune system comes to the rescue by killing the clump of cells, but if it is lucky enough not to be detected by the immune system it will settle someplace else in the bloodstream and it will secrete more enzymes to punch a hole through the blood vessels and find a new place to settle, then presto! A new colony emerges and your primary cancer has just metastasized.

So why is this a problem when it comes to surgery? As part of the diagnostic process cancers are almost always biopsied, now just think about that for a moment, imagine for a second that you have a water balloon filled with cancer cells and then imagine sticking a needle into it to get a sample, now without the graphic deflating of the balloon a tumour will keep its shape, but more importantly what has your doctor just done? They have just ruptured the tumours connective tissue and now you have toxic cancer cells coming out of it going all over the place, bypassing all of your body's defences to make sure that what just happened never does.

So how do surgeons surgically remove cancer without spreading it everywhere? They can't! It's on the cellular level! The only way they could do this is if they took a chunk of healthy tissue without rupturing the tumour and in many cases that's exactly what they do. However, the problem remains, the patient's dysfunctional metabolism is the root cause, the tumour is the symptom. My father had one of his lungs removed which included healthy tissue and he got cancer in the other lung, taking the healthy tissue does not work.

Studies have shown that the stress caused by surgery is known to suppress the immune system and promote metastasis, in a study called "*The promotion of tumour metastasis by surgery and stress: Immunological basis and implications for psychoneuroimmunology*" by the Biopsychology Research Unit, Department of Psychology, Tel Aviv University in Israel concluded the following on stress and surgery-induced metastasis.

> *It is concluded: (a) Immunological mechanisms most likely play a role in limiting metastasis in patients with solid tumours. (b) Immunosuppression can be deleterious, especially when surgery is conducted early before the tumour develops insurmountable mechanisms to escape immune destruction. (c) The most sensitive period for the establishment of metastases is the immediate aftermath of surgery.*

If you have ever been diagnosed with cancer like my father then you will know that if surgery is an option then they will try to get you under the knife ASAP once a diagnosis has been made. People have been rushed into surgery as soon as the next day following a diagnosis which leaves no time for the patient to assess their options or even be told the full consequences of their decisions. The oncologist told my father when he had his lung removed that his cancer was a slow-growing one and that he could have had it for as long as a year before they whipped him into surgery, cut him up and pumped him full of chemo.

That's because most oncologists only tell you what they think you need to know. Many types of cancer take years to develop such as breast and pancreatic cancer. It is said that some can take as long as 10 years or more to develop before it becomes a problem yet the moment your oncologist discovers you have it you are rushed into surgery so fast your feet will barely touch the ground. They don't give you enough time to explore your options because they assume the only ones that work are the big 3. Oncologists who subscribe to this mentality are taking advantage of the fear and desperation of their patients and are bypassing their patient's fundamental right to informed consent, not to mention a violation of the Hippocratic Oath. How can any patient say they were informed when so many are given no time to assess their situation? This is extremely manipulative and predatory behaviour by the medical profession and if you want to see their true colours disagree with them on the big 3 and you will have an experience you won't forget.

Opioid drugs like morphine are considered to be the gold standard of pain relief especially after surgery which depending on the type may leave the patient in chronic to severe pain. However, some studies have linked opioids to tumour progression and metastasis leaving Anesthesiologist's to consider better postoperative pain management options for cancer patients.

In a study done by Patrick Singleton, PhD, assistant professor of medicine at the University of Chicago who the won the award for Best Basic Science Abstract at the Anesthesiology™ 2012 annual meeting, which was called *"The mu-opioid receptor: A new target for cancer therapy?"*. The study discusses how opioids which are substances that act on opioid receptors to produce morphine-like effects in patients, and how they can affect cancer cells and influence cancer progression and metastasis. Dr Singleton and his team including Jonathan Moss, M.D., PhD found that lung cells have 10 times the amount of opioid receptors compared to normal cells and that tumours in mice grew twice as fast when they had the extra mu-opioid receptor and were 20 times more likely to spread.

Professor Singleton said this about the study.

"There is epidemiological evidence to suggest that the type of anaesthesia used during cancer surgery may influence tumour recurrence."

Another study called *"Surgery for Cancer: A Trigger for Metastasis"* by Samer Tohme, MD, Richard L Simmons, MD, and Allan Tsung MD in the Department of Surgery at the University of Pittsburgh's Medical Center, discusses the mechanisms of how surgery has the potential to cause metastasis and reoccurrence of cancer after the procedure, they concluded this with their study:

Metastasis is a common cause of morbidity and mortality in cancer patients. Both experimental and clinical evidence lend support to the idea that surgery which is intended to be a curative option to remove and reduce tumor mass, can paradoxically also augment development of metastases.

Another study called *"Potential impact of invasive surgical procedures on primary tumour growth and metastasis"* by Senior post-doc oncology researcher Maria Alieva, at the Princess Máxima Center for Pediatric Oncology in the Netherlands, examined the potential impact of surgical procedures like biopsy's and resections, which is the partial or full removal of an organ with cancer and the issue of tumour progression. The following is from the beginning of their abstract and the end from their conclusion of the study:

Surgical procedures such as tumor resection and biopsy are still the gold standard for diagnosis and (determination of) treatment of solid tumors, and are prognostically beneficial for patients.

However, growing evidence suggests that even a minor surgical trauma can influence several (patho) physiological processes that might promote postoperative metastatic spread and tumor recurrence. Local effects include tumor seeding and a wound healing response that can promote tumor cell migration, proliferation, differentiation, extracellular matrix remodeling, angiogenesis and extravasation. In addition, local and systemic immunosuppression impairs antitumor immunity and contributes to tumor cell survival. Surgical manipulation of the tumor can result in cancer cell release into the circulation, thus increasing the chance of tumor cell dissemination.

Clinical and preclinical evidence indicate that both biopsies and tumor resections can have multiple effects that stimulate tumor progression, metastatic spreading and outgrowth.

However, given the variety of surgical procedures, tumor types and stages that are encountered in the clinical practice, the conclusions drawn from these studies cannot be generalized.

This study is interesting because it kind of encapsulates the point I have been making throughout this book, without a doubt the study clearly shows that biopsy's and surgery can make cancer worse by spreading or causing reoccurrence, but later it tried to play these risks down by saying the following:

Moreover, the benefit of these surgical procedures for appropriate diagnosis and extended survival is undeniable and outweighs the potential negative effects, advocating against their discontinuation.

So basically what they are saying is that it doesn't matter if they cause seeding or surgery-induced metastases in their patients, as long as they can diagnose what your cancer type is then they can match it with an expensive chemo drug.

I wonder how patients would feel about this considering it's them under the knife, not their doctors.

So is surgery safe? Well, it's not without its risks we know that much. The million-dollar question is, has your doctor told you any of this? Because I would argue that it's pretty important knowing what can happen to you if you go under the knife. In comparison to chemotherapy and radiation, I would say comparatively yes, surgery is the safer option, but personally, this is an issue of informed consent. If you are not made aware of the potential risks before surgery then how does your doctor know what you would be ok with?

Do their special powers extend to mind-reading as well? Like it or not, you are on a needs to know basis with your doctor. I'm not saying that surgery does not have its place, but if you spend a bit of time reading studies on how safe and effective surgery is for your cancer you will quickly realise that surgery causes biological stress, inflammation, suppresses the immune system and can make a tumour spread by causing micro-metastases which are undetectable, and even if it doesn't do all that it could just reoccur where you had it.

The only reason we use surgery today for this type of treatment goes back to the 1800s where the war between the allopath's and imperial doctors were heating up, traditionally both types of medicine were widely accepted and both with very extreme differences in opinion on how disease occurred and how it was treated.

The allopath's which is what all doctors today come from believed that disease was a demon and that it had to be driven out of them by force using brutal treatments like bleeding a person which only made them weak and less able to fight off disease, much like today's approach to cancer. Whereas the imperial's believed that disease came from the body being out of balance and so they used many herbs and natural remedies to restore the body's immune system and treat disease by healing the body. The descendants of the imperial's are essentially today naturopaths and this war on medicine has been going on for hundreds of years.

So when your oncologist recommends surgery for cancer assuming it's even an option I'm sure now you will have a lot more questions to ask, just be prepared for their one size fits all approach and believe me when I say that reading about it here is nothing compared to when you hear it leaving their lips. If you are ever in doubt, which I'm sure you are now, unless your life is immediately threatened, do not feel that time is of the essence until you have all the facts. Remember, doctors are there to give you options and if you don't like these options after thoroughly exploring them then seek alternative advice. Whatever choice you make and regardless of how nice you think your doctor is you are the one that is going through this not them, so make sure you do your due diligence before committing to their advice.

CHEMOTHERAPY

Chemotherapy is the treatment of a disease using chemical substances. If you stuck it out this far I'd say you have evolved enough to know exactly how good chemicals substances are for human health. Chemotherapy has its roots in WWII and was developed in the early 1940s, people who were exposed to cytotoxic chemotherapeutic agents derived from mustard gas were found to have less white blood cells. So a couple of genius pharmacologists by the name of Alfred Gilman and Louis Goodman bumped heads together and thought 1+1 must = 11, so they decided to apply nitrogen mustard's ability to obliterate cells, ALL CELLS, in a lymphoma patient and thus chemotherapy was born.

What gets left out of this mad alchemy is that in the 1920s Rene Caisse was already treating hundreds if not thousands of patients with Essiac using a native American herbal treatment with no side effects whatsoever. Yet since the 1940s chemotherapy has prevailed as one of the leading treatments for all cancer types and has remained largely unchanged until the present day. Chemotherapy today is full of cancer-causing chemicals and getting cancer from this treatment never seems to come up when your oncologist is convincing you to get it. For example:

- **Thiotepa** – also known as Tepadina is a chemo drug used in the treatment of Breast cancer, brain tumours, ovarian cancer, myeloma, Hodgkin lymphoma, High-grade non-Hodgkin lymphoma, leukaemia, Germ cell tumours.

- **Melphalan** - Multiple myeloma, ovarian cancer, neuroblastoma, rhabdomyosarcoma, breast cancer and also used in some conditioning regimens before bone marrow transplant
- **Myleran** - Used to treat chronic myelogenous leukaemia

Here are just a few of the other Alkylating agents in chemo drugs that are known to cause cancer and specifically leukaemia:

- Mechlorethamine
- Chlorambucil
- Cyclophosphamide (Cytoxan®)
- Lomustine (CCNU)
- Carmustine (BCNU)
- Busulfan

These chemicals are listed on the American Cancer Society website so they don't even hide it from you anymore, they are openly telling you that chemotherapy causes cancer, the very thing you're being treated for! So ask yourself, how can any doctor in their right mind think that chemotherapy with these chemicals could successfully heal a person's cancer? It's a recipe for chaos! What's more bizarre is that the most common question asked by patients about chemotherapy is will they lose their hair? When they should be saying, fuck my hair will I lose my life? Hair loss is manageable, loss of life isn't. Chemo drugs are so dangerous that even after being incinerated at 1800 degrees they are still toxic, so how do you think the patient must feel? Not to mention the amount of personal protection needed to make and dispose of the drug, they might as well wear a spacesuit.

There is a long list of short and long term side effects from chemo that oncologists don't tell you and patients don't think to ask. Luckily my father didn't experience pain despite the degree of his cancer, however, this is not the case for many people and the full list of side effects from chemo are alarming.

Short Term Side Effects

Fatigue, hair loss, easy bruising and bleeding, infection, anaemia (low red blood cell counts), nausea and vomiting, appetite changes, constipation, diarrhoea, problems such as sores and pain with swallowing and mouth, tongue, and throat, nerve and muscle problems such as numbness, tingling, and pain, skin and nail changes such as dry skin and colour change, urine and bladder changes and kidney problems, weight changes, mood changes, changes in libido and sexual function.

Long-Term Side Effects

Fertility problems, long term chronic pain, difficulty with focused thinking (sometimes called chemo brain), early menopause, Osteoporosis, liver Damage, heart problems, reduced lung capacity, kidney and urinary problems, nerve problems such as numbness and tingling, bone and joint problems, muscle weakness, anxiety and depression and also secondary cancers.

You ever hear people say that the treatment is worse than the disease? Well, don't people ever wonder that perhaps there is a reason for that? In a paper published in the Australian Journal of clinical oncology called *"The Contribution of Cytotoxic Chemotherapy to 5-year Survival in Adult Malignancies"* by associate professor Graeme Morgan a radiation oncologist at the

Royal North Shore Hospital in Sydney with Professor Robyn Ward and Michael Barton, they concluded the following in the paper:

In this evidence-based analysis, we have estimated that the contribution of curative and adjuvant cytotoxic chemotherapy to 5-year survival in adults is 2.3% in Australia and 2.1% in the USA. These estimates of benefit should be regarded as the upper limit of effectiveness, as some eligible patients do not receive cytotoxic chemotherapy because of age, poor performance status or patient choice.

Also, as noted in the text, the benefit of cytotoxic chemotherapy may have been overestimated for cancers of oesophagus, stomach, rectum, and brain. Even so, any new chemotherapy drug is still promoted as a major breakthrough in the fight against cancer, only to be later rejected without the fanfare that accompanied its arrival.

It is said that in the eyes of big pharma cancer is not a disease it's a business model. For 77 years chemo has been around and look at how far we have come with technology in that time. So why don't we have something even a fraction better than chemo? Because if we did the pharmaceutical industry would lose billions in cancer drugs and has the absolute potential to create global economic chaos. Cancer drugs alone make big pharma more than 200 billion every year and that's a conservative estimate.

In Australia, the average cost of cancer treatment over a lifetime can be as high as $33,400 as of 2008 where the patient may be out of pocket around $5,000. Thank God for Medicare right?

Oh, that's right the taxpayer picks up that bill so in a roundabout way it did cost you!

If you include the additional 145,483 new cancer cases in Australia for 2020 then they have just made more than 4.8 billion dollars over these peoples lifetime. Oncologists are essentially sales agents for big pharma and are incentivised by pharmaceutical companies to give patients chemotherapy. Chemotherapy is the only drug in the market where this incentivised scheme is allowed which proves that many oncologists are acting in the interests of themselves, the hospital they represent and big pharma, not the patient. Oncologists have been busted big time for "flat dosing" that is where they deliberately give you less chemo than the recommended amount so that the hospital makes more money because more chemo is needed to complete a standard course of treatment. In Sydney Australia at the St Vincent's hospital Dr John Grygiel an oncologist was busted for giving his patients 100mg of chemo as opposed to the recommended 200mg to 300mg for his patients. Though I applaud his efforts for giving his patients less poison than the standard dose, the fact is that he and the hospital gained quite the hefty sum as he did this to more than 100 patients. The authorities concluded that he had been doing it for a while and after closer investigations by NSW Chief Cancer Officer David Currow who delayed the release of his findings because he was looking at hundreds of patients going back decades.

In a joint study by Public Health England and Cancer Research UK called *"30-day mortality after systemic anticancer treatment for breast and lung cancer in England: a population-based, observational study"* it details how some hospitals are killing up to 50% of their patients by using chemotherapy and that 8.4% of people who have lung cancer and 2.4% of people who have breast cancer died within 30 days of treatment demonstrating that treatment was the primary cause of death and not cancer. This was a huge study which involved more than 23,000 women with breast cancer and approximately 10,000 men with lung cancer, out of the 9634 Non-Small Cell Lung Cancer men (NSCLC) that had chemotherapy 1,383 died within 30 days indicating that treatment was the cause of death. That means that hospitals are killing as much as 15% of lung cancer patients with chemo where the cause of death is cancer on their death certificate. Breast cancer is one of the most common cancers and has life-altering consequences for many women including hidden long term side effects that are not being discussed by their oncologist. In a study review called *"How breast cancer chemotherapy increases the risk of leukaemia: Thoughts about a case of diffuse large B-cell lymphoma and leukaemia after breast cancer chemotherapy"* by the Department of Radiation Oncology at the Shandong Cancer Hospital and Institute, Shandong University in China, they had this to say about chemotherapy for women with breast cancer:

Breast cancer is one of the most common malignant tumors that have serious impacts on women's health and is often life-threatening. According to statistics published by the World Health Organization International Cancer Research Center, there were approximately 1.38 million new cases of female breast cancer worldwide in 2008, accounting for 22.9% of all female cancers. In addition, 460,000 women died of breast cancer in 2008, accounting for 13.7% of female cancer deaths. With recent progress in neoadjuvant therapy, adjuvant therapy, endocrine therapy and targeted therapy, the survival of breast cancer patients has gradually been prolonged. However, the consequences of overtreatment have also gradually emerged. What should not be ignored are second primary cancers and TRLs (Therapy Related Tumors). In the 1980s, TRL first gained the attention of clinicians. It is a chemotherapy-induced and/or radiation-induced leukemia due to the treatment of primary malignant or non-malignant diseases. Professor Wolff Antonio's latest research has shown that prophylactic chemotherapy or adjuvant chemotherapy for early stage breast cancer patients can increase the risk of TRL. These findings lead us to think that the number of patients who may develop a leukemia triggered by overtreatment cannot be ignored given the large population base of breast cancer patients.

Studies all over the world from United States, England, Canada, Japan, Norway, and Italy have shown that when a cancer patient is in the late stages of their condition that they are prepared to undergo more aggressive treatments which carry higher risks for only a small extension of life. The belief patients have when it comes to chemotherapy is that their oncologist knows what they are doing, and the truth is that oncologists are people first and doctors second, there are a lot of people in the world who are just plain ignorant and doctors are no exception.

The truth is that safer and more effective treatments exist and just because you are not told about them or science doesn't accept them doesn't mean they don't work. Doctors are not educated on what natural treatments can do for us and many will criticize alternative therapies even though they have not studied them. The scientific data used in this book mostly came from doctors and researchers, the same place they get their information when they tell you the big 3 treatments are the answer to your cancer.

When the toxicity of a single treatment can be in your system for more than 12 months I would say that asking the right questions and knowing what you are doing is a no brainer. So before you succumb to the fear tactics used by doctors who rush you into treatment ASAP, do some research on what they are recommending and if you don't like what they are selling you then ask them if they would get the same treatment if they were in the same position? Chemotherapy is not a survivable option in any long-term sense and unless you're lucky enough to be in the 2% of people who will survive beyond 5 years there is still no telling what other long term symptoms may manifest later. We will conclude this section with the wise words of Dr Ralph W Moss PhD a man who has had more than 40 years' experience helping patients deal with cancer, he has even written and edited 12 books and 4 documentaries on questions relating to cancer research and treatment.

"A study was done which shows the majority of oncologists who refer patients for chemotherapy for lung cancer would not themselves take chemotherapy for lung cancer. And in fact if the chemotherapy involved cls-platen, something like 75% of them said they wouldn't take it. But what do these people do all day long? They're sending people for cls-platen."

RADIATION THERAPY

Radiation therapy is the use of concentrated energy particles or waves, like X-rays, gamma rays, electron beams, proton therapy or photon therapy to destroy or damage cancer cells and does this by damaging the DNA within the cell. So how can further damaging the DNA in a cancer cell kill it? Well, that's another reason why it doesn't work and why it presents more problems and side effects than benefits. Radiation is not selective in what cells it kills so it has the absolute potential to turn a healthy cell into a cancer cell. There are three types of radiation Alpha, Beta, and Gamma, where alpha is the least penetrating and Gamma the most, depending on the type of cancer and where it is, this will determine what type of radiation is used in treatment.

Believe it or not, radiation therapy goes back to the 1890s when the discovery of X-rays was first made. After noticing the burns left on people from x-ray exposure doctors began testing it on growths and lesions and it soon became a treatment for diseases such as lupus, rodent ulcer, epithelioma and even tuberculosis. The problem with radiation is that it causes scars, if you have ever seen someone who has been badly burned in a fire then that's what radiation does to your internal tissues. The trouble with scar tissue is that it is very difficult for it to go back to healthy tissue. Now remember when I said that an MRI or a CT scan only detect a tumour if it's a certain size otherwise doctors won't be able to see it, well here is the problem with radiation, it can kill most of the cells in the tumour but it cannot always kill the cancer stem cell, so when your doctor starts to celebrate what a great job they have done it's way too early to determine if the treatment has even worked.

Some of the latest research shows that further damaging the cancer stem cell using radiation makes them tougher and more resilient to kill. In as little as a few months, you could be back at the hospital getting treatment again because your radiation oncologist and radiologist fails to grasp this concept. I don't know why it's so difficult for most cancer doctors to work out, its basic biology that cells have a liquid in them called water, you know H2O, well what happens to water in the microwave when you heat it, it steams or is vaporised, so by water content alone they can shrink a tumour. When they see a size reduction in a tumour they assume that the treatment has had an effect, but all they are doing is killing a whole bunch of daughter cells, not the cancer stem cells. A safer alternative which could produce the same results is to inject bicarb soda in and around the tumour site as suggested and tested successfully by Dr Tullio Siminoichi, an Italian cancer researcher, but I guess that's just crazy talk seeing how bicarb soda is like $2.50 from your local supermarket.

If you want to see what you have to look forward to then google images "radiation treatment burns" and see what radiologists have been putting their patients through in the name of modern treatment. My heart bleeds for these poor women who have been subjected to this disgusting treatment where their entire breast had to be surgically removed because the burns were so bad. There is a whole range of short and long-term side effects from radiation, the short-term ones are almost always nausea, hair loss, fatigue and skin problems. Whereas the long-term side effects could be anything from lung problems to heart problems which can show up years later and when they do they are almost always permanent.

Here are some of the side effects your radiologist probably won't tell you:

Cataract's, fatigue, dry mouth, permanent hair loss, mouth and gum sores, difficulty swallowing, stiffness in the jaw, A type of swelling called lymphedema, tooth decay, problems with thyroid or adrenal glands, infertility, slowed or halted bone growth in children, decreased range of motion in the treated area, skin sensitivity to sun exposure, problems with memory or ability to learn, radiation-induced heart disease and secondary cancers such as skin cancer and leukaemia.

As if radiation treatment wasn't bad enough, I bet you didn't know that you can get high exposure to radiation leading to cancer from your doctor without getting conventional treatment at all. Another diagnostic tool used in the diagnosis of conditions which is a favourite of doctors is called a computed tomography scan better known as a CT scan. The difference between a CT scan and an MRI is that a CT scan uses X-rays (radiation) whereas an MRI uses magnetic fields and radiofrequency pulses to produce pictures of the body's internal structures. A scientific article published by The British Journal of Radiology in 2012 called *"Radiation-induced cancer: A modern view"* discusses how CT scans used in normal doses in the diagnostic stage of treatment may increase the person's risk of cancer, they concluded the following.

There is considerable, though not universal, consensus in the radiation protection community that radiation-induced cancer can occur at the doses and dose rates encountered in diagnostic medical radiation. Although little epidemiological evidence exists for the precise shape of the dose-response curve at *radiation doses <0.15 Gy, mechanistic radiobiological data would support the conceptual canonical theory of a single electron track potentially inducing cancer. Although some theories of radiation risk predict even higher risks at low doses, this LNT model is among the more conservative estimates.*

Another study published in 2013 by the BMJ (formerly the British Medical Journal) an international peer-reviewed journal called *"Cancer risk in 680,000 people exposed to computed tomography scans in childhood or adolescence: data linkage study of 11 million Australians"*, where the objective was to assess the cancer risk in children and adolescents following exposure to low dose ionising radiation from diagnostic CT scans, they concluded the following about the safety and potential risk of CT scans.

Our study is the largest population-based study to date of diagnostic medical radiation exposure. It also provides more information about low dose exposures than was available from the study of Japanese atomic bomb survivors. Our study shows that CT scans during childhood and adolescence are followed by an increase in cancer incidence for all cancers combined and for many individual types of cancer.

So even your doctor's diagnostic tools are causing you cancer. So the question you should be asking yourself now is, if their CT scans can increase the risk of cancer by this much, then how likely is it that you will get better from radiation treatment which uses concentrated doses of it? Also, if you already have cancer and you get multiple CT scans what's to say they are not making it worse? According to these studies that's exactly what they are saying.

I don't want people to misunderstand the point I am trying to make here, am I saying that we have no use for CT scans? Of course not, they are an important diagnostic tool in the medical profession, what I am saying here is, are you informed about the risks associated with multiple CT scans if you already have cancer? This is just another one of those things that doctors feel you don't need to know, because most of them don't know it! The second point I want to make is that if doctors want to use a CT scans to diagnose conditions then so be it, but they must meet two essential criteria before they are used and that is are they safe and effective? What good is a tool if it's effective but not safe? Or safe but not effective? If you are already a cancer patient being treated by your doctor and are subjected to multiple CT scans how exactly are they helping you when they are not even telling you about the risks of what they are doing?

Between the chemo and radiation circulating in a person's body, they become so highly toxic that it can even cause the people around them to feel sick and nauseous. The thought of something like this doing any good to your health is simply delusional, and if you ever want to challenge a doctor or specialist on getting these treatments then ask them to name one biological system or organism on the planet that gets better after you cut, poison and irradiate it? When you see the vacant expression on their face you can probably assume that they don't have an answer, and if they did they are full of shit! This is where peoples blind faith in something can take precedence over their logical brain and get them to agree to a course of action where they are not only misinformed but where their choices have life-altering consequences.

Another study confirming radiation treatment causing secondary cancer which was even described by the researchers as a double-edged sword because it can cause the very thing it's supposed to treat was a review of the scientific literature about radiation treatment and is called *"Radiation-Induced Malignancies Making Radiotherapy a "Two-Edged Sword": A Review of Literature"*. This was done by the Department of Radiotherapy, VMMC & Safdarjung Hospital in New Delhi, India, they concluded the following:

Radiotherapy is an important treatment modality in oncological care. Radiation-induced malignancies (RIMs) are considered as one of the most significant and life-threatening late complications of radiotherapy. A number of general conclusions can be drawn from the discussion in this review.

1) Carcinomas and leukemias are commonly seen in organs receiving low dose radiation; whereas sarcomas are more common in tissues or organ receiving high dose radiation.

2) RIMs are more common with orthovoltage and high Light Energy Transfer (LET) radiations.

3) Children are at higher risk as compared to adults, with chemotherapy and various hereditary disorders increasing the risk.

4) An increased incidence is observed with Intensity-modulated radiation therapy (IMRT) as compared to three-dimensional conformal radiation therapy 3D-CRT due to the dose distribution (larger volume irradiated to lower doses).

Radiation therapy being one of the major treatment modalities of cancer can also sometimes cause cancer, hence truly can be considered a "two-edged sword". RIM is a late and unavoidable side effect of radiotherapy, the exact pathogenesis of which is not well understood. Till date histology of RIM cannot be differentiated from natural occurring tumor.

Another issue that hasn't really been discussed or researched thoroughly is that of Electro-Magnetic Frequencies (EMF). This type of radiation comes from mobiles, tablets, laptops, telecom towers and other android devices. Believe me, when the facts come out about 5G and how this contributes to a person's health over a lifetime these telecom companies are going to shit the bed because 4G was bad enough. Studies have even shown that radiation from sources like Wi-Fi and mobiles can damage the hippocampus in the brain which is responsible for thinking and memory, and why people today seem so stupid. In one study on prenatal rats exposed to radiation from mobiles compared to a control group, it was found that newborns that were exposed to EMF took 3 times longer to complete a maze for a food reward and made twice as many mistakes as the control group.

Mobile devices have shown to cause infertility problems in males because EMF radiation kills sperm, it has also been shown to cause breast cancer in woman and other areas where mobiles are commonly pocketed. Telstra is one of the only telecommunication companies now sending messages to consumers about RF exposure and how to reduce it, and that's because they know exactly what radio frequencies can do to human tissues, particularly the brain in developing children.

Try this, go to your phone in general, then settings, then to devices, then go to legal information and check the information it has on RF radiation. People who use their phone for a call more than 6 mins long increase their radiation exposure to the brain accumulative over a lifetime, which is why it is now law all over the world that all mobile devices be given headsets or earpieces so that it is not kept close to the head. How many people do you know today that are on the phone for less than 6 minutes at a time or with earphones? This may in part explain why so many children that get cancer seem to always get the rare types like brain and blood cancers which could be caused by low exposure regularly over a long period. Let's face it how many parents give their children the Ipad or their phone with the Wi-Fi on just to shut them up? 99.9% I would bet.

The only reason radiation therapy is even used as a main course of treatment has nothing to do with its effectiveness, it has to do with a scientist by the name of Marie Skłodowska Curie, AKA Madame Curie, a naturalized-French physicist and chemist who conducted pioneering research on radioactivity, but was also known for her discoveries with radium and plutonium. In 1903 Madam Curie got a Nobel prize in physics and again in 1911 in chemistry and was a major media junkie who told everyone at the time when X-rays had just been discovered that they would be the easiest way to win the war on cancer. What history doesn't tell you is that in 1902 professor John Beard at the University of Edinburgh first proposed that pancreatic enzymes are the first line of defence against cancer.

Enzymes made by the pancreas which are Proteolytic, amalytic and lypolytic which digest proteins, carbohydrates and fats have an anticancer function other than their primary function which is to break down these foods in the digestive system. He was nominated for a Nobel prize in 1905 in the field of embryology and he spent 20 years of laboratory research which even today holds up to rigorous scientific scrutiny. However, because Professor John Beard did not know how to manipulate the media as well as Madam Curie his research on pancreatic enzymes and cancer for the last 100 years has been largely forgotten. But here's the irony, or what I like to call sweet poetic justice, Madam Curie who crapped on about how great X-rays were to the media, saying that it's the easiest way to treat all cancers and that it was safe died from Aplastic Anaemia caused by overexposure to the X-rays she was recommending we use. Is it just me or do you ever notice how some of the world's smartest people always die from the most stupid shit...

As smart as she was a bit of modesty would have served her well, she may have even lived longer if she hadn't believed that X-rays and radiation was the answer. Today we have carried on her legacy as if to completely disregard all of the warning signs along the way, even though she was completely wrong about radiation as a treatment for cancer. It is neither safe nor effective and the fact that it killed the discoverer and founder of this practice only attest to how naive and ignorant the medical and scientific community can be.

There are many types of radiation that we are exposed to it every day and the long term impact of lifetime exposure is virtually unknown to the public.

The environment has also taken a beating from RF frequencies which are responsible for the massive decline in bee and butterfly populations and also affect some migrating bird species. One study showed how a single mobile device can affect a beehive, several beehives were lined in a row where only a few of them had a mobile device turned on inside, it was concluded that the EMF's seriously impact the bees ability to find its hive, which if it cannot is certain death for that hive. Some scientists and researchers say that if all pollinating insects like bees and butterflies were extinct that humanity would be next, we are that dependant on them.

Another subject not commonly discussed with patients is that of Tumour Lysis Syndrome. This is where the treatment kills a tone of cancer cells and the toxic contents of these cells enter the bloodstream and poison's the patient, that's because the lymph nodes and organs like the liver and the kidneys cannot neutralize the toxins and flush them out of the body fast enough. Yet how many times do you hear these doctors crapping on about how a patient has had a 50% reduction in their tumour? Well, the toxic contents of this tumour which made up the other 50% had to go somewhere, so the question is are they doing more harm than good because patients can die from Tumour Lysis Syndrome.

Hopefully, after reading this you will have some very interesting questions for your radiologist, there is a tone of radiation studies and information for you to get informed so don't just accept the first thing you hear. Like I said before you are the one who has to undergo this treatment, not those who are giving it to you.

GENE & IMMUNO THERAPY

The fourth type of treatment can be either immunotherapy or gene therapy but usually, it's both which are technically different but can be used together, for example, Immunotherapy is where they try to boost your immune system by activating or suppressing it, whereas gene therapy focusses more on the genetic pattern of cancer where they identify the gene responsible then try to repair the damaged DNA within the cell. It can get a bit confusing but the two can be used hand in hand depending on what strategy is used.

There are 3 types of gene therapy, one is to repair damaged DNA within a cell, the other is called gene silencing which is like turning a gene off so it doesn't express a particular quality or function and the final one is to directly kill the cancer cell. It sounds pretty amazing, right? And in some way it is, if only it worked, though gene therapy has the potential to treat many disorders it is still early days and much more research is needed.

The problem with gene therapy in the treatment of cancer like most conventional treatments is that it doesn't work because the whole approach is based on genetics as a cause, which as we established earlier might not be the case at all. The concept of gene therapy first came up in the 1960s and 1970s but it was until September 14th 1990 that it was first used. A young girl was the first person to undergo gene therapy, she suffered from Adenosine Deaminase (ADA) an immune disorder which stops people from being able to fight off infections, people like this are also called bubble babies because they have to live in sterile environments otherwise the slightest cold could kill them. Yet it wasn't until 1989 when it was suggested to be used as a cancer treatment, researchers had teamed up with Dr Steven Rosenburg an American cancer researcher and chief of surgery at the National Cancer Institute in Bethesda, Maryland. It was here when Dr Rosenburg tested how safe and effective gene therapy would be in the treatment of cancer and since then the rest is history.

Unlike chemotherapy and radiation, I won't deny the potential this treatment has but it's still early days, like the other treatments mentioned in this book supported by mainstream science it is not without its risks. One of the problems with gene therapy is that you cannot just shove a gene into DNA like too many clothes in a suitcase for it to repair or silence a gene, it needs a carrier called a vector, this is normally a virus, where the disease-causing agents are removed from the virus and the repair piece of DNA is inserted in its place. However, a possible side effect from this approach is that the virus may recover its ability to cause disease, infecting the patient which is already weak due to their condition and could be life-threatening as many people in this weakened state often succumb to pneumonia.

Another reason why gene therapy doesn't always work is because of how the immune system reacts in the presence of cancer, cancer cells that are about to be attacked by your immune system often develop mechanisms to avoid immune system detection, this is known as "Immunoediting Behaviour". So when gene therapy is introduced to your immune system rather than correcting the damaged DNA, turning off a gene or killing the cancer cell, it may recognise the virus or vector that is carrying it as a foreign invader and kill it before it does what it was designed to. Because these viruses are recognised as foreign invaders and can infect any cell type in the body, the immune system will not only target the virus but also anything it is near. Put simply, it's like a blindfolded kid trying to hit a piñata and instead ends up battering to death his grandmothers fine China. This causes inflammation in the body and in severe cases organ failure which I'm sure you would agree is essential for life. But it gets worse, gene therapy can also cause cancer, viruses can affect multiple cell types so if it does not go where it is supposed to it can damage the DNA in a different cell type and cause other diseases and disorders, if this happens it can occur at the injection site but also anywhere else in the body.

On the 21st of March 2013 on the ABC news Richard Besser did a segment on Medicine which covered a cancer breakthrough, it talked about gene therapy and how it had been used to treat one of their camera crew David Aponte who had suffered from an aggressive type of Leukaemia. Yet despite all the hype and promise of a better tomorrow only 3 months later on the 29th of June 2013 David died in the Memorial Sloan Kettering Hospital, he was only 59. Yet after David's death, there was no mention or retraction of gene therapy being this revolutionary treatment as shown when David was alive despite its utter failure to heal him. I wonder how many people who went on TV promoting a breakthrough cancer drug are still around, especially longer than 5 years, I doubt there would be many...

An issue that never seems to cross doctors minds is the use of immunotherapy after chemotherapy has failed, theoretically, this is a huge contradiction in logic because one treatment (the chemo) is tearing the immune system down while the immunotherapy is trying to at least theoretically, build your immune system up. Why the fuck would an oncologist give you 2 treatments which have the complete opposite effects?

The more you think about this the more you start to realise either A, they have no idea what they are doing or B; you are an experiment to them and this is nothing more than guesswork.

Some of the side effects from gene therapy are fever, colds, vomiting, inflammation, severe chills, drop in blood pressure, nausea and headache which should resolve itself within 24-48 hours. Because the vectors or viruses used can target any cell type and recover their ability to cause disease the disease you can get will depend on what type of virus they used. For example, the herpes virus, if they used this vector on you then you could get herpes as a side effect its that simple. Other side effects could include secondary cancer, this can happen if the DNA was inserted at the wrong spot and results in a solid tumour forming, it has also been known to cause leukaemia.

Gene therapy is permenante genetic modification and is where radiation treatment was in the early 1900s, it's still in its infancy and there is potential for it to work if they can just iron out all the bugs. However, if given the choice between subjecting myself to this treatment with the side effects mentioned a real possibility or eating organic fruit and vegetables and changing my lifestyle then I know which one I would choose. Genetics and biotechnology have interesting potential, but when you look at how we have used them in GMO's and treatments for diseases the cons far outweigh the pros.

I feel we are too primitive to use this technology for cancer treatment and it doesn't help when all the focus is on genetics which even mainstream science admits is poorly understood. I don't know about you but I do not want my food or my DNA altered or tampered with by people who does more guesswork than actual science, even if they did know what they are doing how could we trust what they say is the truth when their data can be manipulated to show exactly what they want us to see?

If you want to see what genetic tampering looks like then google "rainbow coloured fruit" then look at these images and see the kind of genetic tampering I'm talking about, you can get rainbow coloured bananas, strawberries, chillies, oranges, tomatoes and a whole bunch of others, they may look beautiful, but would you trust eating them?

Don't you find it strange that there is not one conventional treatment that doesn't have a side effect that causes cancer? Because I have never heard of anyone getting cancer from eating organic fruit and vegetables? The point is that our ancestors even in ancient times used simple and natural remedies to treat diseases and illnesses and they certainly weren't genetically modifying everything they ate, putting fluoride in their water or vaccinating everyone in their community like we are today. Our ancestors were a lot smarter than we give them credit for and we could learn a lot by looking back if we weren't so focused on rushing forward. We are not the most humble species and we hate to be wrong even if it means lying our asses off to avoid looking stupid in the eyes of other people. Governments and corporations are masters at this, when was the last time you heard a politician admit they were wrong? It never happens...

The mainstream medical and scientific community refuses to acknowledge the power of natural medicine despite the volume of evidence that supports what our ancestors knew all those years ago. Fortunately, today there are also many emerging doctors and researchers that are taking the initiative and bringing us the science that is needed to convince the world that our approach to cancer has been extremely limited and that more diverse personalised therapies based on natural remedies may prove to be the revelation that everyone has been waiting for.

A research team in the UK lead by Professor Dan Bourke and Professor Gerry Potter has researched an enzyme called CIP1B1 which is high in cancer cells but not in normal cells, they said that using salvestrols which are found naturally in many different types of fruit, vegetables and herbs could be an effective means of fighting cancer. It was discovered that when the CIP1B1 enzyme reacts to the salvestrols found in many organic fruits and vegetables that it induces apoptosis, but did not seem to happen from genetically modified fruits and vegetables, only organic sources. Fruits, vegetables and herbs that are bitter or sharp to the taste were also found to have higher amounts of salvestrols, some of these are:

Artichokes, asparagus, watercress, roquette, spinach, pumpkin, olives, currants, apples, rose hips, strawberries, sage, mint, dandelion, plantain, holy thistle, agrimony, vervain and many citrus fruits.

Professor Bourke also said that salvestrols are not produced in plants for our benefit, but is used as a chemical defence from fungal attack on the plants.

Changing your philosophy is paramount to success and when you use the enemies weapons against them and your oncologist cannot answer a simple question, you will begin to see with your own two eyes just how big this lie is. No matter what happens, never sacrifice the truth for politeness and stand up for yourself, do not be intimidated because these people hold degrees, if they cannot explain things to you simply then they don't know what they are talking about.

Hopefully, I have done my job well enough to at least make you stop and think before rushing into treatment as the doctor would have you. The Imperials who used herbs and natural remedies to promote the body's natural defences had it right in the beginning but were taken out by tyrants sole bent on greed, power and control.

The 3 families responsible for this mess are the Rockefellers, Carnegie's and Morgan's who financed the entire medical profession and controls everything from what doctors learn at university, to the industry regulators, to the pharmaceutical industry, and is without a doubt the largest monopoly in the world. These families just happen to be the ruling elite and are worth more than a trillion dollars for each family. We need to change the way we think and stop believing everything in our textbooks like they are gospel and do some thinking of our own, we need to go back to imperialistic medicine or even Ayurvedic medicine which goes back more than 5000 years.

If you or someone you know has cancer always educate yourself before you speak to a doctor because their script is predictable and they cannot recommend a treatment they have not been trained in even if it has the potential to heal you. Just remember that you have other options other than the big 3, so if you or someone you know has cancer don't succumb to their philosophy of CUT… POISON… BURN…

PART V

CHAPTER 14: 7 THINGS FOR AMAZING RESULTS

On April 1st 2014 my father began his chemotherapy for the final time, he had agreed to be re-trialled on the same drug as before despite how utterly useless it was. However, after the radiologist suggested he get another cycle of radiation with chemotherapy my mother took something I said on board for once and asked them about the long term side effects which were never discussed the first time. Seeing the obvious change in his behaviour my mother wanted to know exactly what it could do to him if he agreed to it. They said that it could cause scar tissue on his heart and brain which can lead to several long term issues and that's if it didn't kill him, this was one of those things where unless you ask you are never told the whole story.

From early April till late October he had completed 6 cycles of chemotherapy and by January 2015 we were given the speech again. It was at the point where I would prefer a smiley face sticker than hearing them talk because these doctors had the attention span of a moth when it came to logic and reason. I had unfortunately seen the ending of this predictable play and tried to prepare myself as best as I could. My father was in the clear and he took that to mean that changing nothing was necessary because I was wrong and he was right, I said to him do you know that a single treatment of chemo can be in your body for a year and you have had dozens! Problems began to develop between my mother and father, my mother finally realising that many of the things that I had said were all coming true and in the end she gave him a choice, she wanted him to change his attitude and lifestyle or move out because none of us could take it anymore.

He chose to move out as opposed to changing himself and all of us had felt as if he had chosen his ignorant, destructive lifestyle over his family, a selfish act indeed. By moving out he finally qualified for some money at Centrelink and his brother Paul set him up in a unit in a small town called Terang where my uncle lived, by being close to him he could keep an eye on him in case anything happened. In August of that year, my mother got a phone call from my uncle saying that my father was back in the hospital. He had been sitting in his chair at home when he suddenly collapsed, after hitting the floor he spent the whole night there because he couldn't move, something had gone terribly wrong. At some point, he managed to get to the phone and call my uncle, when he spoke over the phone my uncle knew something was wrong by the way he sounded. My uncle went over to get him and could see something had happened, he was taken to Warrnambool Hospital and after a few tests, they found that his lung cancer had metastasised. His cancer had spread to his pancreas, kidneys, lymph nodes and he also had 10 separate lesions on the brain affecting his speech, thinking, memory and mobility.

When I heard about this I said to my mother "we should go get him and bring him back home", my exact words to her were, "I don't care how you do it, even if you have to lie to get him discharged, he cannot get anymore treatment". My thoughts at the time were if he has another round of chemo it could easily kill him, the oncologist overseeing his treatment at the hospital had organized another round without consulting my mother and was due to give it to him on the 1st of September. My mother and sister agreed to go get him, so for the next 4 hours driving to the hospital, I spent that time telling her why she has to have him discharged no matter what they tell her.

After 4 hours of debates and argument's we arrived at the hospital, my head was pounding from listening to my mother and sisters bullshit which was based on nothing, worthless opinions that weren't even valid because they never tried to understand anything I mentioned to them in the last 5 years. We parked the car and went up to his room, as I walked through the door and he was sitting in a chair in a cold room with nothing but his underwear and a t-shirt, while the oncologist was sitting on the bed talking to him. He was so thin that I had never seen a person's thigh that thin before, he was nothing more than skin and bone. I had learned that just before we got to the hospital that they had given him chemo without consulting my mother which seriously pissed me off. Though my parents were still married they didn't live together, but even so we were his family, I don't give a fuck what the laws are! It was morally and ethically wrong. Sometime after this I sent an FOI request which revealed that the oncologists own notes state that he is in a state of confusion about what is happening, so how could he be of sound mind to make or understand these medical choices?

As I walked into the room I heard the oncologist say to my father "Alan we are going to do radiation on your brain" and when he responded all he could say was "yeah", really slow and drawn out as a child would. My blood was boiling and it took everything I had and more not to explode in a rage against this woman, thoughts of pumping her full of chemo a radiating her brain filled my head, the way I saw it, I couldn't fuck her up any worse, this woman was poison and didn't belong in a hospital.

My mother, sister, uncle and his wife came in just after and when he turned his head to look at us you could tell that it took a few seconds for him to realise who we were, his mental state took us all back because none of us expected him to as bad as he was. When my father realised who we were, he began to cry, it was the first time in my whole life I had ever seen him cry. When the oncologist left I told my mother that they wanted to radiate his brain and I said if you allow this to happen it will kill him or worse turn him into a vegetable. Later when the oncologist had come back she had told my mother and the rest of us what I had overheard. She wanted to do radiation on his brain because the lesions on his brain were her biggest concern. Finally, my mother was starting to get the picture, she asked the oncologist if she thought it would help? The oncologist said probably not, but we can try…GUESSWORK!!! It was sounding more and more like a blind experiment by the minute where my father was the primary test subject, no useful advice came from her at this point and all we heard was the same recommendations, the big 3. My mother said no to the radiation and that she just wanted to take him home, the oncologist refused to listen to her and instead she kept asking my father what he wanted to do which was completely insane because the man had 10 lesions on his brain and in her own words could barely walk or talk let alone comprehend what was being said to him.

Between 2010 to 2015 when I had taken my father to the hospital for treatment I saw first hand how incompetent they were, but I had never met an oncologist as oblivious to her surrounds as this one. For over an hour there was a debate on whether to discharge him or not and she refused to let him go without a fight, my mother said: "Cancer patients are not supposed to have radiation more than once and he has already had it for his condition". Score 1 for Lorraine because she was absolutley right. The oncologist's response to this left me completely and utterly blown away! To this day I will never forget it! She said that she didn't know he had radiation before because she hadn't read his medical file yet, but she had already given him chemotherapy...

After much debate, she had finally agreed to discharge him and we were told to get him the next day, we went back to my uncle's place and stayed the night, but I hardly slept knowing that he was in a hospital with a woman like that overseeing his medical care, it was very unnerving. I realised it was crunch time and that I had to apply as much of what I learned in the last 5 years as possible, I ordered about $500 worth of health foods, supplements and herbs to help his recovery and said to my mother that I don't need any arguments or debates from anyone, we do this my way because you have been listening to doctors for the last 5 years and look at where it has gotten him. The next morning came and I was anxious to leave, my mother and sister were in the hospital doing his discharge while I was in the underground car park putting him in the car, while I was doing it I saw the oncologist from the day before and I wouldn't be lying if I said that the thought of running her over hadn't crossed my mind. I came to my senses quickly when I realised that if I did run her over then the last place I would want to do it is in a hospital where she could be saved. We began our 4-hour journey home and I was eager to put in to practice what I had learned in the last 5 years and prove to my whole family that it can be done, assuming it wasn't too late.

We have covered a lot so far but from here on out we are going to get into the remedies for REAL cancer treatment and what you can start doing right now to give yourself the best chance. Don't worry about remembering all of the details in this book, the details and science are there to explain why we are doing what we need to do and how it can impact certain cancer types. A complete list of cancer friendly foods are mentioned on **page 368** and the detoxification summary is on **page 372**. So let's begin with 7 things everyone with cancer can do right now!

7 Things for Amazing Results

In this chapter, we will look at some of the things that I have picked up over the years which have been shown to improve your health by removing toxins and clearing out your system. It's important to keep in mind that what is offered here are healthy choices and that I cannot guarantee a cure for cancer or any disease for that matter, I can only educate and pass on what I have learned through my experience. The irony is that your doctor or specialist cannot guarantee it either, what I can do is share some of the things I gave my father when he came home and also some of the things I have personally tried with him and researched to be effective with no harmful side effects.

If possible I would recommend asking your doctor to do a complete screen for heavy metal and chemical toxicity on your bloodwork, you would think this would be standard practice but it is not. If anything is elevated above normal then you may be able to pinpoint what you are exposing yourself to and causing your illness. If I recall this may take some time and might be expensive so ask your doctor what the process is and hopefully they will accommodate our request. If not then the following cleanses will get the ball rolling even without the results.

Remember, each cancer is different so depending on the type of cancer the approach will vary. Try looking at your condition as something that needs to be approached from multiple angles, not something where a magic mushroom is a cure-all. So let's begin with fasting.

1. FASTING

Most people think of fasting as a religious practice and others believe it to be counter-intuitive, after all, if you don't eat you die, right? But what if people are eating too much, and that the key to a long life and good health is eating less? Religion has conditioned some people into thinking that fasting is a way for people to suffer as certain religious figures did in the past. In the Muslim faith, fasting is the period known as Ramadan and is a period of spiritual self-reflection and increased devotion towards the teachings of Islam, some of these teachings are to show compassion for those less fortunate than yourself and why all Muslims appear at their place of worship as equals regardless of who they are in the world. I always thought this was a beautiful way to bring people together as equals and show compassion and understanding for those who are less fortunate by putting themselves into the shoes of others for some time and experience what they must experience. Fasting can be traced back to ancient times and was practised by nearly all ancient cultures for good health and wellbeing. Fasting was also used to treat disease and it is where the word breakfast comes from because you "break the fast" by eating.

Fasting gives your body a chance to essentially catch up, particularly your liver which is a real workhorse for your health, your liver secretes enzymes that help neutralize harmful toxins in your food so if you are constantly eating it never gets a chance to rest which can lead to a whole range of medical complaints later in life.

Fasting gives your liver the time it needs to recover and focus its energy on tasks like proper digestion and filling your gallbladder with bile.

Fasting also promotes potent metabolic changes in the body like ketogenesis, stress resistance, lipolysis and autophagy. It has even been shown to be as effective as clinically approved drugs, in fact, in animal studies fasting was shown to reduce the impact of chemotherapeutic agents in mice.

In a study called *"Fasting vs dietary restriction in cellular protection and cancer treatment: From model organisms to patients"* at the Andrus Gerontology Center, Department of Biological Sciences and Norris Cancer Center at the University of Southern California, Los Angeles. They make an interesting point about the effectiveness of fasting and how it contradicts what oncologists and the hospital dietician tells you before you get treatment, which is to eat as much as you can to increase your calorie and protein intake, this is what they said in the first 3 sentences of their Abstract.

The dietary recommendation for cancer patients receiving chemotherapy, as described by the American Cancer Society, is to increase calorie and protein intake. Yet, in simple organisms, mice, and humans, fasting–no calorie intake–induces a wide range of changes associated with cellular protection, which would be difficult to achieve even with a cocktail of potent drugs. In mammals, the protective effect of fasting is mediated, in part, by an over 50% reduction in glucose and insulin-like growth factor 1 (IGF-I) levels.

Fasting has also been shown to increase life expectancy in animal studies and by reducing food intake by 30% in bacteria, worms, spiders, monkey's, mice, rats and many other types of organisms that their life expectancy also increased by 30%, indicating that when food isn't always available in the environment that these adaptations may have developed as a kind of stress response to limited resources. When it comes to cancer many studies suggest that fasting in humans may have just as potent an effect on cancer as chemotherapy without the toxic side effects, though so far these have only been confirmed in mice studies, with our DNA 95% identical to the common mouse it's highly probable that it would work just as well on humans. Studies in rats and mice have also shown that fasting has less neurodegenerative potential and fewer symptoms in neuro disorders like Alzheimer, Parkinson's and Huntington's disease. One of the main things fasting does is that it gets rid of glucose which is exactly what you want if you have cancer.

The benefits of fasting are:

Reduce cholesterol, detoxify the body, weight loss, increased awareness, removes brain fog, reduces inflammation, increases energy levels, dampens the effect of seizures and seizure-associated brain damage, Rheumatoid arthritis, extends life expectancy by delaying age, may reduce the risk of diabetes, can help improve eating patterns, can reduce oxidative damage and even prevent and help treat cancer.

So what is the best fast for you? There are heaps of variations for fasting out there, but intermittent fasting is the one I like the best because it fits in better with my lifestyle. For this type of fast, you should not be eating anything for 12-24 hours and you don't have to do this every day to get the benefits, 3 to 4 days in a row should be fine. For this fast, simply get up in the morning and wait till 1 pm to have breakfast, then eat as much fruit and vegetables as you like till 6 pm. Aim to get at least 8 hours sleep and for the remaining time drink only water or black tea with no sugar or milk, green tea is best for additional health benefits.

No matter what fast you choose just about all of them have a greater effect if you combine the fast with exercise. Fasting will take some getting used to, especially if your addiction is food and let's not kid ourselves, food is awesome! Who doesn't love food and all of its glorious combinations? If you want to kill a few birds in one stone then do your exercise out in the sun for 30min a day and drink only water with this fast and aim to do it 3-4 times a week. I know it may seem counter-intuitive to eat nothing to beat cancer but I have yet to read the book or study that says how to beat cancer by eating cake and biscuits, otherwise that's what I would have suggested.

2. DETOXIFICATION

Detoxification starts with restricting substances that are causing you to be toxic; there are several cleanses that you will need to do to get things working, especially if you have already had conventional treatment.

I recall helping my father get into the bath after he had chemotherapy because he was too weak to do it on his own and the smell of chemo coming through his skin was out of this world! I remember thinking if it's making me feel like this how the hell does he feel? Conventional treatment is massively taxing on the body which is why we are aiming for a full body cleanse and detox program that will get you on the road to recovery.

The following cleanses are a summary of how to clear out your system to get things moving and there's a good chance that one of these areas is specific to the type of cancer you have, so it's vitally important that care is taken when detoxifying these areas.

- **Skin Detox** – The skin is the largest organ in the body so we will need to clear it out so new toxins can be passed through effectively.
- **Colon Cleanse** – Faecal matter can be glue-like due to poor diet and stick to the intestine creating a shopping list of digestive complaints, it is also where the microbes in your gut do their best work to keep you healthy and boost your immune system.
- **Bacteria in the Gut** – Once the colon cleanse has been done we will want to put back the good bacteria so your bowel movement can return to normal and also help restore the immune system.
- **Liver & Gallbladder Cleanse** - The liver is your body's filter and the gallbladder houses the bile needed for proper digestion, the healthy food eaten will not be properly digested if the liver isn't functioning properly. (Do not use a liver flush if you have liver cancer this could be fatal).

- **Parasite Cleanse** – Parasites are more than just ticks and worms they include microbes as well, some have been known to cause cancer so we must clear out any potential freeloaders and restore the immune system.
- **Chemical & Heavy Metal Cleanse** – This is why I suggested earlier that bloodwork be done to determine if there is a high concentration of a specific chemical or metal in your body. Today with all of the toxicity around no one is completely chemical or metal-free so reducing their impact on the body is the purpose of this cleanse.

During your detox program, your diet should consist of all the fruits, vegetables, nuts, seeds, fungi and seafood's that have been mentioned in this book, I am sure there are many more that have not been mentioned so as long as there is no sugar, processed foods, meat or dairy you can't go wrong. Something to keep an eye on while you are doing this is the colour of your urine and your bowl movements. When someone has had chemotherapy or are highly toxic you can expect the colour of their urine to be quite dark, it could be a combination of the body trying to remove toxins and dehydration which is a dangerous combination in any recovering patient. Medications are also known to change urine colour so you will want to monitor the colour of your urine and bowel movements regularly to gauge if what you are doing is helping.

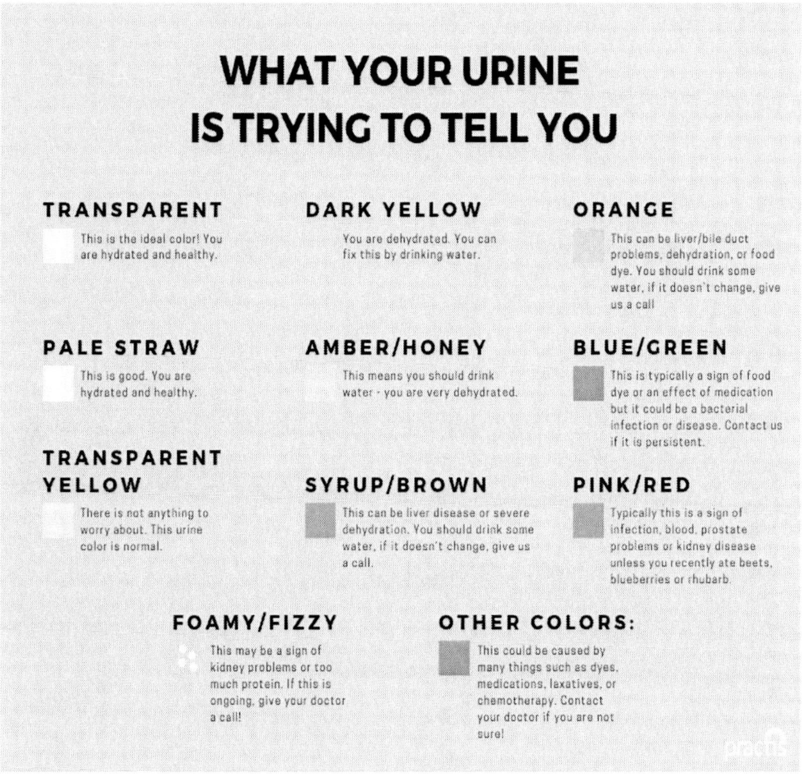

The following cleanses are highly recommended by Dr Edward Group who is also known as Dr Detox and has studied detoxification and disease for more than 15 years, he is one of a great many people credited with helping those with all sorts of diseases and sickness resulting from toxicity. He has also been warning and educating people of some of the health dangers mentioned here in this book particularly that of GMO's in the human diet. He recommends the following cleanses in this order, but there are many variations of these cleanses out there so be sure that they do not conflict with any medications or do not present you any immediate danger.

Skin Detox - Baths Not Showers

For this type of detox, you should add 2 cups of sea salt and 2 cups of bicarb soda, have this bath as hot as you can stand and try to stay in for about 45 mins, when the bathwater cools this is where the toxins will leech out of the skin so do not add more hot water, always towel dry and do not rinse your body afterwards.

This is perfect for purging toxins from the skin, the skin is the largest organ in the body so if you are unable to move around and get yourself sweating then this will help you greatly in reducing your toxic load. It is probably best to have a salt and bicarb bath after exercise because sweating opens the pores and will allow for a greater detox. Instead of a shower use daily bathing like this to stay clean, you can add aromatherapeutic oils to the water for additional health benefits.

Use a salt and bicarb bath at the end of the day because it will probably make you tired, it is also a great way to prepare your mind and body for sleep, sleeping well in a warm, soothing and comfortable environment is essential for cell recovery and is critical for the immune system to do its best work.

Other types of detox baths are a normal baking soda bath, Epsom salt bath, Apple Cider Vinegar bath, Hydrogen peroxide bath and Herbal baths.

Colon Cleanse

This is the first cleanse you should be doing and should be done every day for the first week at least. A simple and affordable way to cleanse the colon is to buy distilled water at the supermarket or use a distiller at home if you have one.

Then, get your hands on to some raw non-pasteurised organic apple cider vinegar, organic lemons and Aloe Vera juice which can all be found in the health food section of the supermarket. You will also need some oxy-powder which is a natural colon cleanser from a good chemist or health food store. Oxy-powder releases a timed controlled oxygen reaction into the intestines that helps to break down and remove the “shit” stuck to the inside of your intestinal tract, thus allowing you to clear and pass waste more efficiently.

Mix 2 litres of distilled water with the oxy-powder and follow the instructions on the back, then add 4 tablespoons of organic apple cider vinegar and add the juice of one organic lemon and 1 ounce of Aloe Vera juice. This is a slight variation on Dr Group's colon cleanse, I have tried this myself and it’s not too bad on the pallet. If you are unable to get oxy-powder then try drinking apple cider vinegar, lemon juice and Aloe Vera like this once a day for at least a month, it will take longer to get the same results plus these 3 ingredients on their own can help the body fight off cancer so it cannot harm.

Children and old people may be more difficult as they are known for being fussy eaters so they won’t be impressed with the taste. You could try using organic apple juice which will improve the taste considerably but only use it sparingly, although organic apple juice has a huge cleansing effect on the body it is also high in fructose which we want to avoid, so use your best judgement.

The Power of Bacteria

Bacteria is one of those things that can make or break you; some studies indicate that we are 10% human and 90% microbial which includes bacteria, which means that the average human has more than 100 trillion microbes in their body. This is where the power of probiotics comes in and I cannot stress the importance of healthy gut bacteria, these are the good guys that break down waste products and help stop the bad ones from moving in and taking over. Probiotics have been known to help with all sorts of problems associated with the GI tract, they can boost your immune system, give you vitamin B6, B12 & K2, prevent irritable bowel syndrome (IBS) & several types of diarrhoea, C-diff infection, ulcerative colitis, necrotizing enterocolitis, eczema, vaginitis, pouchitis, Crohn's disease and strengthen gut mucosa, so there handy little buggers to have around.

By week two the GI tract and colon should start to improve so we need to put back the good bacteria that your poor diet, antibiotics or chemotherapy has killed. These microbes in your gut also need to be fed the right food, you wouldn't give your goldfish pepper instead of fish food, unless your me when I was 5. All vegetables are fair game but the best ones are the dark leafy greens so that is what you should be feeding them, try thinking of it like looking after a pet.

Diseases like cancer often start in the intestinal tract and that is where you need to concentrate your efforts, GMO's damage your intestine and the insecticide on GMO's kills the good bugs in your gut, so try to get a good quality broad-spectrum probiotic, inner health plus seems to work well.

Go to your chemist and try to get a probiotic with the most variety, not the highest amount because what you need is a diverse range of bacteria doing different tasks for you. Also on a final note do not take Yakult for a probiotic, don't get me wrong I love the stuff and I think I'm the only one who wishes they made that flavour an actual drink, but for our purposes here it only contains the *Lactobacillus casei* Shirota strain and its high in sugar which is a big no-no for cancer.

Liver & Gallbladder Cleanse

The liver is your bodies filter, so it makes sense that if the filter is dirty and clogged then your body will be too, the liver is the only regenerative organ in the body and is the most metabolically complex of all organs even the brain. The liver performs more than 500 functions in the body so it works bloody hard to keep you alive. The liver is tasked with fighting off infections, helping the blood clot, neutralizing toxins, manufacturing proteins and hormones, controlling blood sugar, and at any one time, the liver can hold as much as 10% of your body's total blood. A fatty congested liver means you probably have liver stones, the gallstones you get don't come from the gallbladder they are produced in the liver after years of alcohol abuse and a bad diet. Studies done by Dr Edward Group showed that most people over the age of 30 have a highly toxic liver, symptoms include:

Fatigue, abdominal bloating, hormone disruptions, increased cholesterol, skin conditions, loss of appetite, allergies, poor memory, mood swings, trouble digesting fats, sleep disorders and many more.

For someone with cancer or whose health is in a fragile state particularly after chemotherapy there may be an increased danger to doing a full-blown liver flush, that's because when your liver detoxifies your body it releases these stones which are highly toxic along with other toxins stored in fat which is deposited into the bloodstream. This increase in toxicity with chemotherapy could result in organ failure and possibly kill someone. However, these toxins cannot stay in the body they must be purged slowly and regularly, this is done by eliminating the toxins going into the body and maximising those that go out with minimal risk to the person.

There are 2 ways to cleanse the liver and detoxify the body. There is a full-on flush and a gradual cleanse, so depending on your state of health and what type of cancer you have you will need to think carefully about which one you do.

The flush was the progenitor idea from the author and researcher Andreas Moritz who wrote the book "The Amazing Liver and Gallbladder Flush", and in his own words removed more than 3000 liver stones from his liver treating a whole range of problems that he suffered from his whole life. He also wrote a book on cancer called "Cancer is not a disease it's a Survival Mechanism". Until recently I didn't realise how valuable his work was until it fixed an issue I've had for more than 18 months. I used the flush in his book and after a week my right side rib pain had completely gone. Even my energy and mental alertness increased and I felt like I had the energy I did when I was a kid.

You will need to eventually remove as many of these stones as you can to restore the functionality of your liver. Below is what they look like.

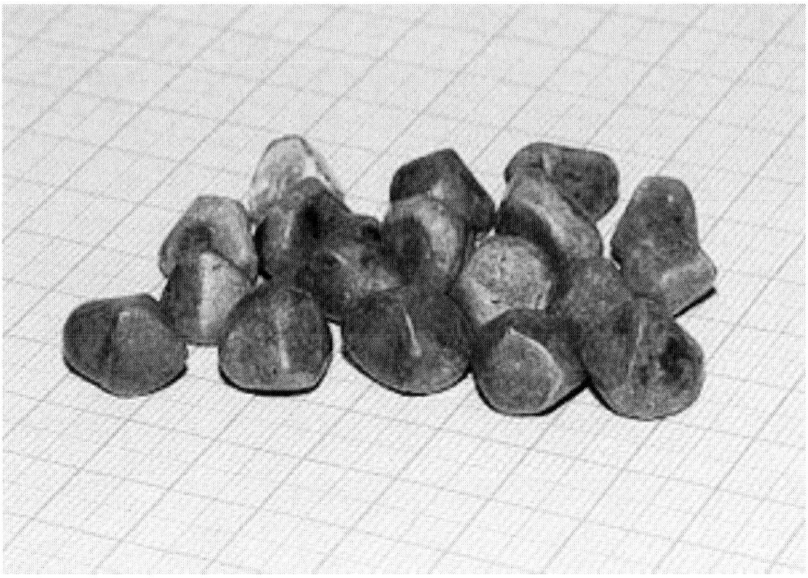

For copyright reasons I cannot tell you the details of the flush to help you rid yourself of these stones, but you can get the book on Amazon for about $15 which is worth its weight in gold.

A safer option for those not able to do the flush is a slow detox, this is done by getting some malic acid tablets from the chemist which will soften the stones in your liver, take these as instructed on the bottle. Then you will want to drink dandelion and lemon tea with a milk thistle supplement first thing in the morning and before bedtime on an empty stomach. It may take longer to achieve the same results but it is safer for those in a fragile state.

Parasite Cleanse

Parasites are not just ticks and worms they are also microbes like bacteria, viruses, moulds and yeast which make up to 20% of all known cancers, so this has to be on our list as a course of action. Symptoms of a parasitic infection can range from depression, stomach pain, unexplained weight gain or loss, diarrhoea, nausea, vomiting and a whole range of other symptoms depending on the parasite. Parasites are known for giving very non-specific symptoms which could appear like a whole range of other chronic medical issues, this is also why 9 times out of 10 your doctor sends you packing not even thinking parasitic infection. Parasites like tapeworms have been known to live in people for as long as 30 years and can grow more than 82 feet long, that's 30 meters! Surgeons have even found a shit load of them "literally" during colonoscopies, so parasites can be a huge problem.

Because the symptoms are so generic, it's not always clear that someone has a parasitic infection and parasites like tapeworms go straight under the radar because there is no test other than a colonoscopy to detect them. So unless you want a 30m monster rolling around in your intestines or some microscopic blood-sucking parasite draining the life out of you, you will need to do something to remove any potential parasitic infections. There are 2 options here, you can buy a parasite cleanse in pill form, one recommended is Paratrex. It was created by Dr Edward Group himself which you can buy on his website www.globalhealingcenter.com. I have never tried it myself and you could just as easily go to your local chemist and ask for their best parasitic cleanse. I have heard that Paratrex has excellent results, but it's a bit pricy if you are on a budget.

You should be able to pick up a decent parasite cleanse for $25-$50 at your local chemist.

When it comes to parasites and general health I would even go the extra mile and dice 2 cloves of garlic and leave it for 15 mins to react with the air, raw garlic contains allicin which has been used throughout history for boosting the immune system, treating illness, fighting infections and reducing inflammation, it also has antiseptic and antimicrobial properties which makes it a powerful medicine. The use of garlic like this goes back for centuries and was used by the Egyptians, Greeks, Babylonians, Romans and the Chinese. Even if you have a common cold, doing this with some Manuka honey on a teaspoon and adding ground cinnamon with a couple of cloves works wonders. I'm not a complete barbarian so if you cannot eat raw garlic on its own then make some vegetables together and get it into your diet once you break your fasting. By week four you should be using the parasite cleanse as instructed, many foods have antimicrobial properties so you will want to eat them as part of your new diet. Some of these are:

Garlic, Ginger, Pumpkin seeds, Coconut (Fresh), Apricots, Wormwood, Cucumber, Pomegranate, Onions, Pineapple (fresh, not tinned), Raspberry and Watermelon.

Chemical and Heavy Metal Cleanse

People are exposed to heavy metals and chemicals every single day and because they are known to hang around for years it may take a bit of patience and persistence to get them out. Fortunately, it doesn't take long to get the ball rolling once the body starts to function properly, these cleanse's are things that everyone should be doing as a preventative measure if they have some type of chronic illness. This is why earlier I said if you can get a blood test done it may indicate a possible cause, however, some heavy metals that could be causing problems and not normally tested for are copper, zinc, aluminium, and thallium, and some tests can be very expensive which may not be practical for those on a budget. So here is what you can do to get them out.

Bentonite Clay – Good old-fashioned mud, who would have thought? Believe it or not, clay has been used for thousands of years for a whole range of medical problems. It is high in most minerals that the body needs and even has anti-inflammatory properties, the minerals that are in bentonite clay are also alkalising which is perfect for balancing the pH level in the person's body. Due to the nature of clay which is quite sticky, it works by going through your system by binding and sticking to toxic chemicals & heavy metals, even harmful bacteria and parasites get stuck, which then gets flushed out of your system when you have a bowel movement. You ideally want to eat bentonite clay on an empty stomach either first thing in the morning or just before bed.

Ideally, you are after organic food-grade bentonite clay which can cost up to $100 so you will have to shop around. If you go back to the old day's humans ate a lot of dirt, this occurred when food wasn't washed properly and the soils were richer and healthier giving us their minerals and good microbes, whereas today most food is chemically treated. A great combination to try is to mix bentonite clay, activated charcoal and cilantro or coriander for a more complete cleanse. According to Robert C Atkins MD. Eating approximately 400mg of coriander per day will remove most heavy metal toxins in 2 weeks, which is amazing to think about in terms of results.

Some foods have been known to remove heavy metals in the body, particularly those high in Pectin which is what is used in jams to give them their thickness, and are typically found in the rinds of fruits and vegetables. The best sources are green apples, cabbage, bananas, beets, grapes, carrots and the pith of citrus fruits. Coriander can cross the blood-brain barrier and remove heavy metals that get into the brain like mercury, lead and aluminium.

There are a few things to keep in mind with bentonite clay, some say you can take it every day and others say not too. I found that when I took it for more than 4 days in a row, it gave me a headache. That said it's perfectly fine to use bentonite clay, but you must know your limits, if you suffer from any of the below symptoms stop immediately and wait a couple of days before you continue.

Some of the possible side effects are:

Head Pain, Nausea, Fatigue (Eeoyre) *or extreme energy* (Tiger), *Body aches, Nasal or sinus issues, Sore throat, GI irregularities, Cold Sores, Skin Rashes, Sleeping difficulty, Increased or decreased sex drive and Flu-like symptoms.*

Note: It's important to understand that these side effect won't exactly be from the clay itself but the toxins that it is pulling from your body, so if you get these symptoms after taking bentonite clay you must stop and listen to your body.

If you have cancer you may already have these symptoms so monitor your reaction carefully after taking this, take a couple of hours after medications and preferably on an empty stomach. Bentonite clay attracts heavy metals so do not use a metal spoon or anything metallic, use a wooden spoon to mix the solution before you drink.

We have finally completed the overview of these cleanses, and so from here, we are going to look at a few more things that need to be understood about cancer and health in general.

3. Anti-Inflammatories

Inflammation is the bodies attempt at self-protection and throughout all stages of cancer inflammation is present, that's because much of the world today is a pro-inflammatory lifestyle. Professor Bharat B Aggarwal, at the Department of Bio-immunotherapy at the University of Texas, discovered a molecule called Tumour Necrosis Factor or TNF, which was discovered to be an anti-cancer agent and one of the major mediators of inflammation, but he also describes it as a double edge sword. TNF used in the right way can stop cancer growth by reducing inflammation, but if you have a poor diet then TNF can allow cancer to grow without interference, and to switch TNF back on to anti-cancer mode something as simple as Turmeric could the job.

Long-term chronic inflammation can lead to multiple diseases and not just cancer; it has been linked to multiple sclerosis, asthma, rheumatoid arthritis, stroke, heart attack, cardiovascular disease, diabetes and many more. Inflammation is the body's response to foreign invaders such as chemicals, metals, viruses, bacteria, fungus and things like free radicals. White blood cells are sent to the affected area to deal with the invader which may result in warmth, redness and pain depending on the severity. The trouble with cancer patients and the TNF superfamily, which is a whole range of anticancer molecules, is that they don't work because the conditions are not right for them to do so. It's like pulling the wire out of a light switch and wondering why nothing happens, but if you give your body what it needs it's like putting the wire back in.

Pro-Inflammatory Foods to Avoid

Sugar, All fast foods, Junk foods, Dairy, Grain Fed Meat, Refined Grains, Bad oils such as Vegetable oils (corn, soy and canola), all hydrogenated or partially hydrogenated oil and avoid all deep-fried foods.

Anti-Inflammatory Foods

- **Vegetables** – Most vegetables, specifically Peppers (All), Broccoli, Collard Greens, Spinach, Kale
- **Fruits** - Berries, All Citrus, Tomatoes, Avocados, Cherries, Grapes, Pineapple
- **Meat** - Oily fish like Salmon, Mackerel, Tuna, Cod and Sardines, look for mercury-free and pole caught and not fish caught by a dredge.
- **Nuts** – All unsalted nuts
- **Mushrooms** – All mushrooms are fair game
- **Spices** - Turmeric, Black Pepper, Cloves, Ginger, Parsley, Sage, Rosemary and many more...
- **Oils** – Olive, Coconut, Ginger, Clove, Tyme, Rose, Fennel
- **Seaweeds** – All edible varieties like dulse

This is just a snapshot of some of the foods you might have around the home. If you are looking for an eating plan around an anti-inflammatory diet then try the Mediterranean diet which consists of these types of foods.

4. Acidity vs Alkalinity

Studies have been done on acidity and alkalinity and their relationship to cancer for ages. It was found that every cancer patient is in a more acidic state than alkaline. The pH scale ranges from 0-14 and the pH in the blood and the body is constantly being adjusted based on the foods we eat, below 7 means you are in an acidic range, whereas above 7 you are in an alkaline range with the ideal range for humans being 7.5.

Below is a picture of the pH scale so you can better understand the range of acidity vs alkalinity.

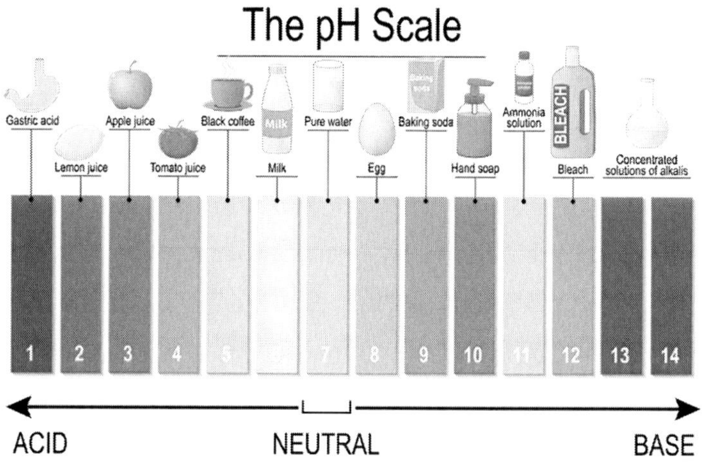

So how do we regulate our bodies so that we are in the correct pH range? If you have cancer then you already know that you are in an acidic state, so the simple answer is to be more aware of the things that are making you more acidic. Do not be fooled into thinking that the lemon, apple or tomatoes in the pH image will increase your blood acidity, they are only acidic before they are digested. After they are metabolized they form alkaline bonds which will make your urine more alkaline. Fermentation occurs when the body is forced to replace the normal method of energy production which is oxygen and glucose, for a more inefficient method creating build-ups of lactic acid and other acids. Dr Otto Warburg a biochemist and two-time Nobel Prize winner said the following on cancer and acidity.

"All normal cells have an absolute requirement for oxygen, but cancer cells can live without oxygen – a rule without exception. "Deprive a cell 35% of its oxygen for 48 hours, and it may become cancerous."

Dr Warburg has made it clear that one of the root causes of cancer is oxygen deficiency, he is also the one who discovered that cancer cells are anaerobic, which means that they do not breathe oxygen, and cannot survive in the presence of high oxygen levels which are found in people who have a pH range above 7. This research goes back to the 1930s, that's how long doctors have been sitting on this information while they were treating patients with pro-inflammatory drugs like chemotherapy. So what can you do to make your blood more alkaline? Blood acidity is not to be confused with gut acidity, the gut should be highly acidic so it can properly break down your food, the blood should be in the pH range of 7.5.

Here are 3 easy ways to change your blood acidity to the correct range.

- Use bicarb soda. Add 1/8 tbsp (600 mg) of bicarb soda to an 8 oz. (0.237 litres) glass of water. **Caution:** This has the effect of changing the pH of your gut, do not do it every day, only once a week in conjunction with the second and third method.
- Use lemons in your drinking water. Lemons are anionic so when you drink lemon water your body reacts with the anionic properties of the lemon making the water alkaline as your body digests it. OR
- You can buy pH drops and use them in your water.

Putting oxygen into the blood it vital and is why hyperbaric oxygen therapy could be used as a cancer treatment in combination with other alternative approaches, this concept is well understood by oncologists yet it is rarely if ever suggested as a course of treatment despite the obvious biology of cancer in the presence of oxygen.

5. Gluththione (GSH) – The Master Antioxidant

This is the master antioxidant and detoxifier for your cells, more than 117,000 peer-reviewed scientific studies have looked at this molecule and the majority have concluded that people are sufficiently deficient. Italian researchers from the Department of Experimental Medicine in the Section of General Pathology in Genoa, have found that people who are deficient in GSH have oxidative stress which may be a contributing factor to the development of cancer and neurological disorders. Glutathione is by far the most important antioxidant in the body, it prevents cellular damage by free radicals and peroxides and it even plays a role in supporting apoptosis in cancer.

Glutathione is produced by your body so you must give your body what it needs to create and use this wonder molecule.

Foods that contain a high source of glutathione are:

Milk Thistle, Green apples, Cabbage, Carrots, Cilantro (Coriander), Grapes, Free Range Eggs (Preferably Raw), Garlic (Raw), Brazil Nuts, Arugula, Berries – Strawberries, Raspberries, Blackberries and Blueberries, Bok Choy, Red & Green Peppers, Citrus fruits, Broccoli, Brussel Sprouts, Cabbage, Cauliflower, Collard Greens, Kale, Mustard greens, Radish, Turnip, Watercress, Pinto beans, Garbanzo beans (chickpeas), Pinto beans, Lentils, Spinach, Asparagus, Avocado, Beets and Black-eyed peas.

6. Exercise

Exercising has been proven to boost the immune system and to help pump fresh blood to the capillaries around the body, so lying around all day is not going to carry those anti-cancer nutrients to where they need to go. Studies have shown that exercising can lower cholesterol, reduce the risk of type 2 diabetes, lose weight, reduce the risk of heart disease, improve the strength of your bones, muscles and joints and can also leave you feeling with more energy, better mood, improved sleep and there are even some anti-cancer benefits.

Exercise should be done daily even if you have to pace up and down the house just to get you moving about and sweating, if you're so weak that getting to the top of your stairs is an effort then that should be your daily goal until your strength increases. If you can move around freely then go for a walk outside in the sun and kill 2 birds with 1 stone. If you are too weak or bedridden, then get one of those hand grips, or do leg raises where you rest, even some stretching exercises can get the blood flowing so trying touching your toes if you are in a lethargic state. There are many approaches to getting your blood circulating, you may even try yoga or Tai Chi, both of which have huge benefits to mind body and spirit. If you don't think either of these could work for you than just remind yourself, that's your old life talking, so maybe now is the time to change. Another idea for improved blood flow is to treat yourself to an incredibly relaxing massage, it relieves stress and increases blood flow to the whole body, so consider this if you get stuck for choices.

7. Sunlight and Vitamin D

For fuck sake go outside! I know its the digital age but there is a whole world out there waiting to be experienced. The production of vitamin D from natural sunlight is so important in boosting the immune system that it really cannot be substituted with a tanning bed or Vitamin D pills. Also known as sunlight vitamin D, there are many health benefits to daily exposure which include a reduction in inflammation, improves brain function, lowers high blood pressure, improves muscle function and some studies show that it can even protect against cancer, heart disease and neurodegenerative diseases.

Cancer patients in chronic to acute pain may have no choice if they are bedridden, my father was so weak that going outside was a 30 min process, so I know it's easier said than done. A minimum of 30 minutes per day in summer and 45 mins in winter is more than you'll need each day and do not put sunscreen on, when you're finished just go back inside. If getting outside and moving around is too difficult then you can get Vitamin D supplements to fill the gaps, but as I said, nothing compares to real sunlight on your skin.

So now that we have covered the 7 things that everyone with cancer should be doing, we will now take a look at some things that science has found to have a direct impact on solid tumours and blood cancers like Leukaemia.

CHAPTER 15: EATING CANCER TO DEATH

In this chapter, we are going to cover some of the most important foods in cancer prevention and what you can use to treat specific types of cancer. In a Ted X talk by Dr William Li titled "Can we eat to starve cancer", he mentions the role of angiogenesis in cancer patients and how it is a common denominator in all types of cancer. The talk is centered on the idea that by eating certain foods you can prevent angiogenesis from happening and starve cancer from its blood supply. His talk and what many people have been saying about beating cancer by eating healthy is supported by a Harvard study on 79,000 men which Dr Li talks about in his presentation, whereby consuming cooked tomatoes twice a week decreased the angiogenesis in prostate cancer after diagnosis. These men were also less likely to develop more aggressive types of cancer from replacing animal fats with plant fats from foods like avocadoes, walnuts, soybean, canola, and olive oils. So you are about to learn exactly what is in our food and what it can do for us without the use of synthetic drugs.

Salt

All salt's are not created equal. Our bodies have an electrical charge which is essential to our survival; electricity sends signals to the brain, keeps our hearts beating and helps with our normal metabolic functions in our day to day life. According to Dr Leonard Coldwell if you eat standard table salt it essentially cuts the inside of your arteries resulting in small haemorrhages which your body sends cholesterol to fix the bleeding.

That's because standard table salt is made up of an anti-caking agent comprised of Silic or Silicon which is essentially sand. In some countries like France, 35% of their table salt even has fluoride compounds such as sodium or potassium fluoride. Sea salt is much healthier than standard table salt, however, these days with so much pollution in the sea this too is a growing concern.

What you are after is Himalayan pink salt which is by far the healthiest salt on the market. This type of salt should be your main dietary salt which helps to make up the bulk of chloride in our bodies, chloride also aids the production of hydrochloric acid for our digestive system so we can break our food down properly and get the nutrients our body needs. According to Dr Mercola, 85% of Himalayan pink salt is sodium chloride which is pure salt and the remaining 15% has 84 trace elements and minerals that our body needs. Himalayan pink salt can be a bit pricey, but a large grinder will last quite a while. On a final note, do not use this salt for salt baths, it can be quite expensive and if your detox bathing every day it's going to add up so use sea salt instead.

Seafood

We all know that fish is good for us, it is packed with omega 3 fatty acids which the body cannot produce and must come from an external source. Fish has been known to help prevent heart disease, reduce the risk of Alzheimer's, boost brain development, ease depression, improve your skin and hair, is the only good dietary source of vitamin D, it can prevent asthma in children, reduce the risk of autoimmune diseases like type 1 diabetes, improve sleep quality, and even help with cancer.

All fish and shellfish are an excellent source of protein and essential fats, however, some caution is needed when buying certain types of seafood from your local supermarket or your favourite sushi shop. For example, most people don't know that the Salmon they buy from these places is not organic or pole caught, and are probability pellet fed. The red colour of salmon, for example, is artificial, salmon flesh is white or greyish in appearance, the red colour happens when fish are fed synthetic pellets which have everything from chicken feathers, animal offcuts, organs, blood, and Astaxanthin. Astaxanthin is essentially a dye where fish farmers can choose what colour they want the flesh of their fish to look like; it is a synthetic chemical that is structurally identical to what fish would be getting if they were eating crustaceans in the wild. Again if you have any concern about what is in your food do your research. Four corners did a program on Salmon farming in Tasmania by a company called Tassal. Tassal like most big corporations only cared about their quarterly statement and have little regard for the massive damage these salmon farms are causing to the environment, it is also significantly impacting the health of the fish they are farming and the people who eat them.

This is what happens when corporations adopt the philosophy of profit over the planet, so buyer beware. Also eating younger fish is healthier than older fish especially flake which is a gummy shark, the older the fish is the more mercury it accumulates and I don't need to tell you how dangerous that is.

Seaweeds

Seaweeds are probably one of the most overlooked nutritional sources of food in the world, they contain anywhere between 10 – 20 times (depending on the species) more minerals than land-based plants and have anti-inflammatory, anti-microbial, anti-fungal and anti-cancer properties. These are a must in the cancer patient diet, so try to add them where you can.

Sodium alginate is a compound present in all seaweeds and is brilliant for removing heavy metals and toxins like the ones found in chemotherapy and can also help the thyroid recover from exposure to radiation treatment.

Seaweeds can bind to toxins and turn them into salts which can then be excreted through the skin during sweating or your daily detox bathing. Seaweeds contain a full spectrum of beta-carotene, enzymes, amino acids, fibre, octacosanol and tissue oxygenation. Seaweeds also promote the following:

Cell development and nerve function, they are 20% protein, have EFA's, good for breast and urine fibroids, prostate inflammation and adrenal exhaustion. They can boost the immune system, stimulate white blood cells, have powerful anti-oxidants, has high levels of magnesium, calcium, iron and vitamin D. They also have high levels of iodine which are essential to recovery after radiation treatment by nourishing the thyroid gland and the adrenals, sea kelp can improve eye conditions, lower cholesterol, lessen stretch marks, chronic fatigue, help with symptoms of HIV, herpes, menopause and chlamydia.

Kelp

This is something that you could go to any beach around the world and find so it's only natural that it would be at the top of the list. Kelp is a blood purifier, great for swelling lymph nodes, help to support intestinal flora, detoxification, antioxidant, reduce the effects of radiation exposure, cholesterol, artery plaque, increases energy levels, helps the heart, nerves, glands, hormones, immune system, allergies, can help to dissolve solid tumours, reduces an enlarged prostate, bowel soother, laxative, toxin remover, and aid in irregularities in the colon.

There are literally hundreds of seaweeds you could choose from that taste great and are nutritious. Some of the species to keep an eye out for are:

Nori or purple laver (Porphyra spp.), Aonori or green laver (Monostroma spp. And Enteromorpha spp.), Kombu or haidai (Laminaria japonica), Wakame, quandai-cai (Undariapinnatifida), Hiziki (Hizikiafusiforme), and finally Mozuku (Cladosiphonokamuranus).

You may have to do a little digging to get your hands on some of these but you can always ask your local Asian grocery store and see what they can offer you. You can always forage seaweeds yourself which is free and in bulk, this is a perfect option for those on a budget and increasing your knowledge of wild edibles.

Marine Phytoplankton

Marine phytoplankton is an enzyme that's active because it is alive. It contains every known mineral and all amino acids that our bodies need for optimum health and is more powerful than fish or flax oil and is the original source of Omega 3.

Little digestion is needed as it has high levels of chlorophyll which detoxify the liver and digestive tract, increases oxygen intake, fuels muscles for higher endurance and recovery. It is also good for the brain, immunity, antifungal, antiviral, antioxidant, improved circulation, heart function, allergy and asthma relief, and an instant useable source of energy. This would be a great supplement for any cancer patient and if your budget allows it. It's also worth using it to reduce and remove the toxic effects of chemotherapy and radiation treatment if you have already had them.

Vegetables

The list of useful and nutritious vegetables are endless, but how many of us eat them? I mean the organic ones that are chemical and GMO free? With our busy lives always on the go who has the time or the money to consider these options and buy organic. It doesn't help to know that good quality food is more expensive and is less accessible than GMO produce and don't even get me started on whether it's fresh or not. The supermarket isn't completely useless, and you will be able to get a regular fix of some of your favourites, but for those you can't, I'd recommend your local farmers markets or growing your own. There are tonnes of vegetables that are great for us and nutritiously dense which also have anti-cancer properties such as broccoli, collard greens, and bakchoi.

We don't think of garlic as a vegetable in its own right rather than an ingredient to improve the flavour of other dishes, but raw garlic is probably the number 1 anti-cancer vegetable you could have. The top 10 anti-cancer vegetables to incorporate into your daily diet are:

Garlic, Broccoli, Bak Choi, Chillies and peppers, Onions, Brussel sprouts, Cabbage & especially purple cabbage, Beets, Kale and Tomatoes preferably cooked.

You can find Organic tomatoes tinned at the supermarket but fresh is always better. All of these vegetables have been known to have a direct or indirect effect on cancer so getting any of them into your daily diet cannot harm you. There are so many vegetables to choose from its crazy, you cannot go hungry nor can you get sick by eating vegetables. There are heaps of scientific studies out there that show how good vegetables are and they are packed with antioxidants, essential vitamins and minerals and all the building blocks the body needs to heal, so develop a taste for them. **See Page (362)**

Fruit

Fruits are a tricky subject in cancer treatment because the concept of starving cancer involves restricting your sugars which fruit clearly has. Technically speaking all fruit is fair game but you will want to limit your intake to all the citrus and berry fruits like lemons, limes, oranges, strawberries, raspberries, blackberries, blueberries and also apples. These types of fruits are nutrient high compared to their sugar content so these are the ones you should consider eating most of the time. They are full of vitamins and antioxidants and are relatively cheap to buy at your local supermarket, you should be able to get organic berries in the frozen food section for around $10 that can easily be stretched out over a week so the cost isn't too bad. Believe it or not, some people live entirely on fruit and nothing else, we call these people fruitarians and the most famous one that I know of was Mahatma Gandhi, so if it was good for Gandhi it can't be too bad for you.

Magic Mushrooms

Mushrooms are powerful medicine and perfect for treating cancer and I'm not talking about the ones some people use to expand their minds, the mushrooms I'm referring to have another power, and that is their ability to shrink tumours. There have been many studies over the years on mushrooms and their ability to activate the cancer-killing cells in our body to prevent future breakouts; they also have antiviral and tumour shrinking abilities. Japan who has traditionally used a wide variety of mushrooms in their cuisine also happens to have one of the lowest cancer incidence rates in the world.

A joint study by the Medical Department of Tokyo University the National Cancer Centre Laboratory and the Tokyo College of Pharmacy showed a complete recovery in 90% of guinea pigs injected with cancer cells after eating the Agaricus Blazei Murill mushroom. With results like this, it's no wonder mushrooms are great for cancer, oncologists could only dream of the day they could get a 90% reduction in tumour size using conventional drugs so this is a must.

Your local supermarket may not have the following variety of mushrooms so again get friendly with your local Asian grocery store.

Reishi Mushrooms

This little mushroom packs a punch when it comes to fighting off disease and it has been used all over Asia and traditionally it has been used in Chinese medicine and their cuisine for more than 2000 years! It has been used for boosting the immune system, fighting off viral infections such as the flu (influenza), swine flu, avian flu, lung conditions including asthma and bronchitis, heart disease, high blood pressure, cholesterol, kidney disease, cancer and liver disease. Studies have shown that it not only plays a role in tumour reduction but also in preventing metastasis in primary cancer.

If you can get your hands on Reishi mushrooms here's what to do for maximum results. Add the mushrooms to a large pot of water and bring to a boil, once boiled turn the heat down to a gentle simmer and leave for at least 2 hours, anything less and you will not be able to get the full effect of this mushroom. The Tea or stock from this mushroom is what you are after which should have a golden brown colour, try drinking it hot like tea or if you cannot stand the flavour add the stock to a soup to improve the taste.

Maitake Mushrooms

The Maitake mushroom is said to have similar properties to the Reishi Mushroom, associate professor of urology Sensuke Konno at New York Medical College, showed that the active ingredients in Maitake and Maitake extract combined with

Vitamin C not only reduced bladder cancer cells by 90% but did so in as little as 72 HOURS!

Mushrooms like the Maitake are also good at preventing angiogenesis, most of the exotic mushrooms mentioned here seem to possess that unique ability.

Shiitake Mushrooms

Some studies indicate that this mushroom may play a role in fighting off cancer, a polysaccharide (a sugar) found in the Shiitake called Lentinan may not kill cancer cells directly but may boost several aspects of the immune system inhibiting tumour growth.

A study done in 2006 and published in the Journal of Alternative and Complementary Medicine showed that ethyl acetate found in shiitake mushrooms could induce apoptosis in two cell lines of breast carcinoma, one non-malignant breast epithelial cell line and two myeloma cell lines. Though many scientists in the community are in two minds about the effectiveness of Shiitake as a cancer treatment its nutritional value cannot be denied, it has Niacin, Pantothenic Acid, Vitamin B6, Riboflavin, Manganese, Phosphorus, Selenium, Copper, Zinc, Potassium, Magnesium, Vitamin D and Iron, making it a diverse and powerful medicine for the recovering cancer patient.

White Button Mushrooms – These mushrooms are delicious, high in vitamins, minerals and amino acids essential for good health, but unfortunately there are no known anti-cancer properties of the button mushroom other than a healthy source of vitamins and minerals. Still, there is no reason why you cannot eat this as a part of your diet, though the anticancer effects are unknown that's not to say that it doesn't have something to offer like its exotic relatives if not a healthy source of nutrition.

These mushrooms are just some of the many exotic mushrooms with medicinal properties and why Chinese medicine uses more than 100 different types of mushrooms for all sorts of conditions, yet one thing is clear, you cannot exclude mushrooms in a recovering cancer diet, they are potent and powerful healers.

Nuts

Nuts are high in unsaturated fats vitamins and minerals; studies show that regular consumption of nuts like walnuts, almonds, Brazil nuts, peanuts, and pecans can help prevent many health issues and cancer is one of them. Some nuts like walnuts and pecans are super high in antioxidants which are perfect for reducing oxidative stress. Here are a few nuts that have been shown to affect cancer.

Walnuts

A study led by Professor Elaine Hardman at Marshall's Joan C. Edwards School of Medicine showed mice that ate a regular diet of walnuts could reduce breast cancer by up to 50%, and when cancer did occur it grew 50% less than the control group. Walnuts are extremely high in antioxidants 25 walnuts have as much as 8g of Vitamin C which is equivalent to 100 oranges. In another animal study called "*walnuts have the potential for cancer prevention and treatment in mice*", also done by Professor Hardman she concluded that walnuts have multiple ingredients that could act by multiple pathways to contribute to the suppression of developing cancer.

Almonds

Almonds are a great source of unsaturated fats; they are high in Vitamin E, copper, iron, calcium, manganese, magnesium, riboflavin, phosphorus, fibre, phytosterols, vitamins & minerals, antioxidants and are also known to help prevent cardiovascular heart disease.

Almonds have also been shown to prevent breast cancer, in one study done by the University of Colima in Mexico it was shown that regular high consumption of peanuts, walnuts, and almonds proved to be a protective factor against breast cancer by a factor of 2-3 times, but did not show this effect when the consumption was moderate to low. Almond oil also has many health benefits; it's an anti-inflammatory, boosts the immune system, has anti-hepatotoxicity effects and can also play a role in the reduction of colonic cancer.

Brazil Nuts

Brazil nuts are one of the highest known sources of selenium which is an antioxidant and trace element particularly hard to get in sufficient quantity from most foods. Brazil nuts can help with thyroid function, can improve the function of vitamin C & E, fortify the immune system, aids healthy fetus development, reduce the effects of cold sores and shingles and also help fight off viral infections. But most impressively in 1998, a study by health professionals at Harvard collected nail samples from 33,737 men between age 40 and 75, though Selenium supplementation was not given to them the nail clippings were used to measure their intake of Selenium in their normal diet.

After 6 years it was concluded that men with the highest selenium in their diet had a 65% lower incidence of prostate cancer and that daily consumption of 159 micrograms would prove to be a protective measure. Another health study by Harvard which started in 1982, collected blood samples from 14,916 American doctors who were healthy, concluded 13 years later that men with the highest Blood Selenium levels had a 48% lower incidence of advanced prostate cancer.

So in a nutshell, nuts are definitely worth incorporating into your diet whether you have cancer or not, I realise that many people suffer from nut allergies these days and if that is the case then I don't need to tell you to avoid nuts in recovery. There are plenty of other foods you can be eating daily to make up your diet, but if you have breast, prostate and colon cancer or any cancer of the gastrointestinal tract, then get these in your diet.

The great thing about brazil nuts, walnuts, pecans and almonds is that they taste great, and they are perfect for satisfying cravings because they are quite filling, personally when I buy all these nuts I mix them all and veg out near the TV. Also, if you are a big meat eater and find yourself craving meat, nuts and mushrooms can be an excellent substitute that leaves you feeling full and satisfied.

Apricot Kernels

The highest natural source of vitamin B17 is Laetrile or Amygdalin, which is found in apricot kernels and also 1400 different plants most of which people eat. There is a lot of controversy around this little kernel and if you look into it well enough you will be astonished at what it is capable of doing, this is also why authorities and Big Pharma have demonised and treated it like a controlled substance. Laetrile is like the holy grail of killing cancer cells; it works in such an efficient way that oncologists could only dream of recommending something so effective. It works like this...

There are two enzymes present in all cancer patients

- **Rhodanese** – which is an enzyme found in all cells EXCEPT for cancer cells.
- **Beta-Glucosidase** - which is an enzyme found ONLY in and around cancer cells

Cancer is such a hog for sugar like glucose, it absorbs the glucose in the B17, but the cancer cell doesn't have the enzyme Rhodanese to neutralize it, cancer cells have Beta-Glucosidase instead, which unlocks the Benzaldehyde, glucose and the cyanide which is bound together, once the enzyme breaks them apart it allows the Hydrogen cyanide to selectively poison the cancer cell and leave healthy cells unharmed. Laetrile is essentially a smart bomb for cancer cells, and because our healthy cells contain Rhodanese the excess B17 is converted into a natural painkiller like aspirin, perfect for those who have symptoms of pain.

Authorities have demonised apricot kernels as a cancer treatment and have put them on par with illegal drugs like meth and cocaine. The Food and Drug Administration in the US has made its use in any form illegal and have even used fear labelling like here in Australia which is designed to discourage its use. A professional arm wrestler by the name of Jason Bail was sent to a maximum-security prison and was looking at more than 20 years jail with bail set at 1 million dollars for selling apricot kernels online after he successfully treated his terminal cancer which was the size of a grapefruit. The argument that landed him in jail was that he said it was a "miracle cure" for cancer and that the FDA claimed that he cannot say it's a cure because there is no medical science to prove his claim. As if the FDA would ever get an unbiased study on it... The media then pumped the fear of cyanide poisoning into people and completely disregarded the fact that not only did he save his own life where conventional treatment had failed him but probably saved the lives of his customers.

Another victim of this mentality is Dr Cal Streeter D.O family practitioner, speaker and author of "A Doctor Goes To Prison" where similar events take place. To summarise what the book is about, he describes his experience dealing with the FDA as extremely troublesome especially when they imprisoned him for successfully treating his terminal patients by using apricot kernels. But the FDA claimed that the results didn't matter because he did not use an FDA approved drug-like chemotherapy which would have killed them.

I have personally tried apricot kernels even though the bag had a warning saying do not consume I knew that they were 100%

organic so I decided to try it for myself. The warning on the bag was regarding cyanide poisoning which is what all of the fuss and fear is over. I was having 10 a day for close to a month till I finished the bag and had absolutely no side effects what so ever, I even gave a small handful to my dog after I noticed a growth about 5cm x 5cm showing through her coat. My reasoning for this was, if she can eat her own shit everyday and live to 11 then this should put a skip in her step. I guess even the dog knew intuitively that it was good for her and probably a pleasant change from the birdseed infested crap she had been eating all her life. All I know for sure is that after a month or so the lump on her side got soft and even shrunk to the point where it was no longer visible through her coat. I can't say with 100% certainty that it was because of what I did but I had no other explanation, so I put the result down to food for thought!

I did learn that in northern India, on the border of China and Afghanistan deep in the Himalayas there is a primitive tribe called the Hunza and these remarkable people could teach us a lot about health and longevity. There are virtually no diseases found in their tribe of 30,000 and are said to be extremely happy and healthy people. They don't eat much meat and they grow organic food with no pesticides, they are largely cut off from society and are kept to themselves, yet amazingly it is not uncommon for males to father children into their 90's and those that do look as if they are 40.

But it gets even better, it is also not uncommon for people to live to 100 and many people from their tribe have been known to live even longer, to maintain this lifestyle they eat plenty of raw fruit and vegetables and a favourite of theirs just happens to be apricot kernels.

The Hunza who are traditional apricot farmers can eat between 30-50 kernels a day, so I'm not suggesting you rush out and buy a bag and stuff your face just because the Hunza do, I am merely pointing you in the right direction so that you can decide if this approach is something you want to do. Personally, the taste is what I can only describe as chemical cherry, and if you eat several at once, your tongue may go numb as the taste is very strong.

Supplements or foods that can help support B17 absorption and its effectiveness is Zinc, which acts as a Laetrile transporter, also Vitamin C, Magnesium, Manganese, Selenium, Vitamin A, Vitamin E, Vitamin B6, Vitamin B9, and Vitamin B12.

Laetrile is best to take on an empty stomach as the digestion of food can interfere with the absorption process, so a couple of hours before or after a meal is best, I took them 3 times a day around breakfast lunch and dinner with no trouble other than the bad taste. The best method I found was to blend the kernels and add freshly squeezed orange juice with a bit of lemon juice in it and shot it like tequila.

Important Information – The FDA in America has banned laetrile and made it illegal to use in pill and liquid form as a treatment for cancer, even the kernels are very hard to get.

It is a safe assumption that everywhere else is the same and for the same reason, I am not recommending this is what you do because legally I can't, I am only reporting on what I have done based on my own experience and what I have researched.

The FDA claims as many other health departments that it is toxic for human consumption but they don't say that when they are pumping you full of chemo or the million other drugs out there on the market. If you buy a bag of organic raw apricot kernels at a health food store you will see the labelling warning you not to eat them, I ignored mine, so for peace of mind if you want to try this approach do your research and don't just take my word for it.

Oils

Oils are such an underrated source of nutrition, health and wellbeing. There are good oils and bad oils, so to begin with we will get the crap out of the way so we can concentrate on the good stuff. The two oils you want to avoid are canola and vegetable oil which are heavily GMO, you may also want to avoid animal oils as well for the reasons mentioned earlier in dairy and meat. Oils can be used for so many beneficial things, from cooking to aromatherapy and over the last few years supermarkets have been diversifying their stock to accommodate the growing interest in organic cooking oils. So here are a few I found to affect cancer.

Organic Extra Virgin Olive Oil

Olive oil is probably the best for cooking and is much healthier than canola, vegetable, and animal-based oils, you can even get butter made out of olive oil called Nuttellex which isn't too bad. Its gluten & dairy-free, low in cholesterol and has nothing artificial, but most importantly it tastes great and should be ok in the cancer diet. Try having a baked potato with Nuttellex butter, salt and pepper and a few other of your favourite vegetables and you won't miss meat at all.

Olive oil contains polyphenols which act as antioxidants and can relieve oxidative stress throughout the body, according to the FDA it is also a heart-healthy monounsaturated fat that they recommend 2 tablespoons a day which could be extremely beneficial to your health. I'm not one to trust the FDA after everything mentioned so far, but other science seems to support this.

Approximately 73% of olive oil is oleic acid which has anti-inflammatory properties and some studies indicate that it may even affect cancer. There is also evidence that suggests that it could also prevent Alzheimer's, heart disease, stroke, type 2 diabetes, anti-cancer properties, antibacterial and may even help with rheumatoid arthritis.

If 2 tablespoons can do all this then, by all means, use to your heart's content. It has also been shown that olive oil is not a cause for obesity so don't worry about putting on an extra few pounds.

Coconut oil

The coconut is also called the fruit of 1000 uses and that's because you can do just about anything with it. The nutritional benefits are also amazing, coconut oil contains fatty acids with potent medicinal properties, it can help to burn fat, kill harmful microorganisms, reduce seizers, raise the good HDL cholesterol, boost brain function in Alzheimer's patients, can nourish the thyroid glands which may be inflamed due to heavy toxins in the body and may also relieve symptoms of hyperthyroidism.

Coconut water is full of electrolytes and can even be substituted for a drip if fluids are down in a survival situation, so the humble coconut found on the beach of our favourite tropical getaway is amazing! Always get organic coconut oil, it can be a bit pricey but it is a very versatile oil to cook and use. You may also want to get organic coconut water, it's a healthy and tasty way of bringing your fluids back up if you have trouble staying hydrated. Coconut water and oil are perfect for those with gastrointestinal issues because it's soothing on the GI tract, the oil can also curve hunger cravings by keeping you fuller longer which means you are less likely to binge on all of your old favourites which are probably not so healthy.

Hemp oil

Good old Ganja! It's no surprise why marijuana is a banned substance, so many studies have been done on the effects of marijuana and cancer and the reason it is not legalized is that the pharmaceutical industry cannot patent a natural plant without genetically modifying it, so now that's exactly what they are trying to do. The oil has been shown to kill skin cancer and many others. The cannabinoids in marijuana have also been effective against Leukaemia and are smoked for their ability to kill pain which can be a common side effect to many cancer types. Cannabinoids are a class of diverse chemicals that affect the cannabinoid receptors in the cells that alter the neurotransmitter release in the brain; this is why it is effective on pain because the signal for pain is disrupted.

A case report I found encapsulates the extent of how far doctors will push toxic therapies on someone just because it is their job, unfortunately, some doctors cannot comprehend the effectiveness of something that is outside of what they have been trained in, and this is perhaps one example in thousands going on all over the world every single day.

A case report in oncology in 2013 called "*Cannabis Extract Treatment for Terminal Acute Lymphoblastic Leukaemia with a Philadelphia Chromosome Mutation*", showed cannabis extract or hemp oil to be particularly effective against the most aggressive type of leukaemia. This was done on a 14-year-old girl who had undergone 34 months of conventional treatment including 10 rounds of radiation to the brain and a bone transplant with regular blood transfusions, and after all of this, it was finally acknowledged by the patient's medical staff that they had failed to treat her cancer. The haematologists and oncologists charted that she has been diagnosed with a terminal malignant disease and that she had been treated to the limits of available therapy, they concluded that in all likelihood that she would die of a stroke in 2 months. Not accepting this the family did what I did with my father, they jumped online and found studies of hemp oil for treating cancers like leukaemia, so in their desperation, they obtained hemp oil from an outside source to achieve the effects mentioned in their research.

Between the 4th to the 20th of February her blast cells had risen from 51,490 to 194,000, which is insanely fast! Hemp oil was given at regular increasing intervals and was mixed with honey to overcome the bitterness, by day 5 which was the 25th of February 2009 her blast cells peaked at 374,000, the next day they had dropped which reflected the increasing dose of hemp oil being administered, they continued to increase the dose and as a result, the girl suffered from nausea and typical euphoric symptoms associated with cannabis. She then developed an infection and was administered to the hospital, due to their regulations they had to limit the dose of hemp oil she was receiving, this slump is reflected in the graph shown in the study, she was later released back home after being administered a heavy antibiotic. Dosing was maintained at 1ml 3 times a day until day 78 more than the projected 2 months survival given by her doctor. She then complained of stomach pain and was readministered to the hospital where they had discovered gastrointestinal bleeding, due to pancolitis (inflammatory bowel disease) a pre-existing condition. But sadly she died, she had passed away due to a bowel perforation.

It was later concluded that before the hemp oil treatment the girl was severely ill, severely underweight and she had endured chemotherapy and radiation treatment for 34 months yet the results on her blasts cells were at acceptable levels after only 20 days. The doctors said that hemp oil has demonstrated anti-proliferative, pro-apoptotic and antiangiogenic properties and that cannabinoids might show selectivity when attacking cancer cells, unlike conventional chemotherapeutic agents which have widespread cytotoxic effects.

They acknowledged that their most advanced chemotherapeutic agents have failed to control the patient's blast cells of which the side effects have ultimately resulted in the patient's death. Whereas cannabinoids had no toxic side effects and with an increasing dose a rise in the patient's vitality was observed.

I found this report sad but also familiar, what this young girl had endured in 34 months was unforgivable, and if doctors had a fucking clue what they were doing then in as little as 20 days she would have been spared the torment and madness that is conventional therapy. This girl had her whole life ahead of her and it was ripped away because of the ignorance of doctors and the greed of corporations.

Yet sadly her situation is not unique, as it is going on all over the word every single day and makes what is known in this book even more necessary.

Clove Oil Extract

Clove has been used in Indian cooking and traditional Ayurveda medicine since ancient times and its anti-cancer properties are noteworthy. Clove oil extract works best on more specific types of cancer and those that would benefit the most would be cancer of the oesophagus and melanomas. A study done by the Institute of Cytology and Preventive Oncology in Noida, India called *the "Comparative anticancer potential of clove (Syzygiumaromaticum)–an Indian spice–against cancer cell lines of various anatomical origin",* found that when 3 different clove oil extracts were taken, 0.1ml, 0.2ml, and 0.3ml (0.3ml is approximately 4.6 drops) the maximum results showed an 80% cell death rate and induced cell membrane rupture in oesophageal cancer cells. The active ingredient in clove is called eugenol which makes up 80 to 95% of clove and is the reason why clove can prevent food from spoiling. It also has antibacterial, anti-fungal and anti-inflammatory properties which help to reduce DNA damage and is also a powerful numbing agent which is why it is still used in dentistry today.

Caution:

Clove is great for many ailments, but like most things too much can be toxic, it can have a cytotoxic effect if used in large amounts, therefore it is best to take in small doses. Do not apply to the skin directly because it will burn and have an exfoliating effect, therefore use another oil to dilute it such as coconut, or olive oil. If you want an aromatherapeutic effect then use essential lavender oil add 1 drop of clove for every 10 drops of other oil and apply to the skin.

If in doubt about how to use it correctly do your research or ask a naturopath for advice. Do not use any cheap oils and only buy organic essential oil.

Frankincense Oil

This is probably one of the most powerful oils you could have in your arsenal. Frankincense oil has anti-cancer properties, it boosts the immune system, fights infections and can even improve mood and relieve anxiety. The compound responsible for these anti-cancer properties is called AKBA which is acetyl-11-keto-beta-boswellic acid. Leading researcher Kamla Al-Salmani at the University of Leicester said that after studying AKBA found in frankincense oil that after a year of research AKBA was shown to kill ovarian cancer even in the late stages with no side effects. There has also been a positive association by using frankincense oil in treating brain, breast, colon, pancreatic, prostate and stomach cancers. Historically, this oil has been used for more than 5000 years and was used to treat a whole range of complaints, it just goes to show you the power of traditional medicine and that just because it is old doesn't mean it doesn't work.

The power of essential oils and their anti-cancer properties cannot be overstated, essential oils and their constituents have potent anti-cancer properties and when used correctly they can be powerful contributors to good health and disease prevention. The only thing that is more impressive than these oils ability to kill cancer cells is that they do so without producing any harmful side effects.

Herbs & Spices

Now I would love nothing more than the 11 secret herbs and spices at KFC to be the answer, but unfortunately, that is just a pipe dream. The herbs and spices mentioned here are by no means the only herbs and spices proven to have a measurable effect on cancer, but these are some of the best in natural cancer treatment and prevention that I have found.

Before jumping into things it's important to note exactly where you get your spices from, most spices are imported which means they get irradiated by quarantine so pests do not enter the country, quarantine also kills many of the anti-cancer properties in the spices we are after so it may be a bit pricey but go to your local health food shop and buy organic local spices if you can. So now that's out of the way let's begin with one of my favourites, ginger.

Ginger

Ginger is one of the worlds most cultivated herbs and was used in ancient history more than 5000 years ago in Greece, the Middle East, Asia and Europe. It was first discovered in south-east China and was a huge favourite of spice traders. Ginger is so powerful and diverse in its uses that it was a component in more than 50% of all traditional remedies and it was said that Confucius never went a meal without it.

In a study called *"Anticancer Effect of Ginger Extract against Pancreatic Cancer Cells Mainly through Reactive Oxygen Species Mediated Autotic Cell Death"*, by the Shimane University Faculty of Medicine in Izumo, Shimane, Japan they concluded the following:

> *The present study demonstrated that the extract of Syussai ginger (SSHE) had potent growth-inhibitory and cell death-inducing activity against pancreatic cancer cells including Panc-1 cells. The extract was also effective under hypoxic conditions, which inevitably develop in all solid tumors to varying degrees and influence the resistance of tumor cells to radiotherapy and conventional chemotherapy. In addition to pancreatic cancer, SSHE also induced a marked cell growth retardation and cell death in a variety of tumor cells, which supports the possibility of applying ginger extract and its active constituents for treating cancers.*

Aside from the anticancer benefits, ginger is so powerful that it can be used to combat the side effects of chemotherapy and radiation which is perfect if you have already had treatment. It can also be used for arthritis, morning sickness during pregnancy, reduces respiratory problems, prevents migraines, prevents blood clots and works great for boosting the immune system and fighting off the common cold.

Turmeric

Turmeric is another cancer-fighting spice with potent anti-inflammatory properties and gets this from the Curcumin or Curcuminoids found within. There have also been more than 6000 clinical studies that show turmeric to be the number one spice to use to heal a whole range of diseases and disorders like cancer.

Turmeric has also been shown to have a positive effect on liver disease, Crohn's disease, arthritis, joint pain, Alzheimer's, Inflammatory Bowel Disease, blood sugar issues like diabetes, anti-microbial issues and cleaning out the arteries, so it's great for people with high cholesterol.

When turmeric is eaten very little of it is absorbed, this is because the liver thinks that it is a foreign substance, so the liver makes the turmeric water-soluble to flush it out of your system. However, a compound found in black pepper called piperine inhibits this process by the liver and a study showed that just a ¼ of a teaspoon was enough for turmeric levels to skyrocket and that the body could absorb 2000 times more Curcumin. The other way for turmeric to be absorbed is to eat it with a plant fat like avocado, nuts or coconut oil, this way curcumin will be absorbed directly into the bloodstream via the lymphatic system which partially bypasses the liver. Some studies even show the potential for this to be complete cancer treatment in itself but admit the bioavailability of the curcumin is better when other spices are added creating a synergism that the individual ingredients would struggle to achieve on their own.

Ginseng

Ginseng was used more than 5000 thousand years ago and was discovered in Manchuria China, though it was thought to be used as a food at the time its medicinal applications came shortly after. America and Canada also had wild ginseng and the commercial exportation of ginseng from Canada to China began in 1716 after a Jesuit priest working among the Iroquois heard of its value in China.

Oddly enough both the Native Americans and the Chinese had independently developed the same uses for Ginseng in their culture and by the 1900s China had exhausted the wild supply of ginseng which the Koreans had grown in response to Chinese demand.

Red ginseng has very potent anti-cancer properties compared to white ginseng and that has to do with the way it is prepared, white ginseng is air-dried whereas red ginseng is either steamed or heated which produces anticancer ginsenosides as a result of the heating process. Red Ginseng can induce apoptosis/paraptosis as well as angiogenesis.

In 2016 in the Chinese Journal of Natural Medicine an article called *"Red Ginseng and Cancer Treatment"*, went on to say the following.

> *The structure-function relationship analysis has revealed that the protopanaxadiol group ginsenosides have more potent effects than the protopanaxatriol group. Sugar molecules in*

ginsenosides inversely impact the antiproliferative potential of these compounds. In addition, ginsenoside stereo selectivity and double bond position also influence the anticancer activity. Future studies should focus on characterizing active red ginseng derivatives as potential anticancer drugs.

Yes, you read that right! Ginseng is so good they could make anti-cancer drugs out of it, so why don't they? It's funny that something like ginseng could be the active ingredient in a drug that your doctor can recommend but not ginseng by itself as it exists naturally, talk about double standards...

Caution!

Though Ginseng is an excellent anti-cancer measure, it has also been known to clash with prescribed medications so before taking this potent cancer killer talk to your doctor about any possible side effects.

There are so many amazing herbs and spices that you can use to fight cancer that you are spoilt for choice, here are a few more that are worth your time.

Black Pepper, Sage, Saffron, Rosemary, Oregano (Authentic Oregano), Dill, Parsley, Flaxseed, Aloe Vera, Burdock, Slippery Elm, Cinnamon and Mistletoe.

By now I hope you realise that there are so many things we could use to heal our bodies instead of synthetic drugs and that your situation is as hopeless as you believe. The takeaway lifestyle that we have become accustomed to may be convenient but it comes at a price. These are just some of the things that I have come across over the years and there is no reason to think that there isn't just as many more.

Already you can see that our scope of available therapies have been severely limited by the powers that be and that if you want your life back then you are going to have to take it because while they are in control you will be at the mercy of the system and we all know exactly where that ends.

CHAPTER 16: HOUSEHOLD WEEDS THAT HEAL

There are 5 common household weeds you will want to get friendly with, which are not only super effective at healing the body but they are everywhere and free of charge. I guarantee that short of living in a desert if you have grass then you will likely have one or more of these growing in your yard which means that free medicine is within your grasp.

When I first learned about foraging for wild plants many of them were unknown to me until I read Markas Rothkranz book "Free food and Medicine", this was critical in me learning the value and importance of what was growing all around me and what most of us go out of our way to kill. However, there is a warning to using plants from around the home, if you have been spraying chemical herbicide, insecticide or fungicide around the house then using the plants mentioned here is seriously inadvisable. Try getting the seeds off them and grow your own in organic soil or find somewhere where you know spraying hasn't occurred, if you are in a hurry then you can always buy them online but educating yourself in these potent healers is something that cannot be bought.

The weeds that are mentioned here are just a few of literally hundreds with just as many healing applications and if you ever go for a walk around your neighbourhood you will be astonished at how many different species are growing in people's front yard. Yet one thing is certain, just as the book is titled you cannot go hungry or in need of medicine with it growing all around you once you know what to look for. So let's begin with one of my favourites the Dandelion.

Dandelion

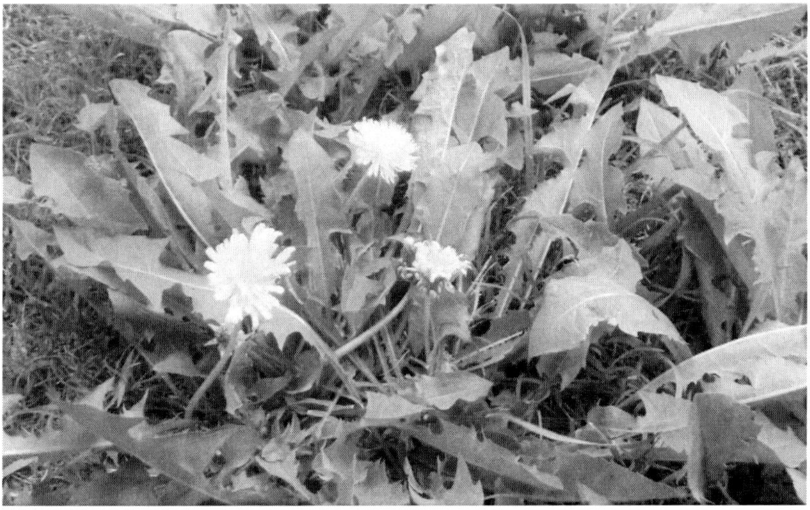

The wonderful dandelion is a favourite among children who pick the stems and blow the seed pods scattering them all over the place in hopes that their wishes come true. Well, sometimes wishes do, at least in the healing potential this plant has to offer. It's unclear where the behaviour of picking dandelions to make a wish came from, perhaps it was a tradition passed down to ensure the widespread continuation of this amazing plant which is part of the lettuce family.

The dandelion is a superfood. The entire plant is edible and is a blood cleanser, kidney cleanser, helps to dissolve kidney stones, improves bowel function, anaemia, cholesterol, prevents cancer, gastrointestinal health, it helps diabetes by managing insulin, its high in vitamin A and E which prevents free radical damage, vitamin C & D, calcium, iron, manganese, magnesium, phosphorus, potassium, sulphur, sodium, saponins, and phytoestrogen.

The young flowers are sweet with a slightly bitter aftertaste and the leaves are pretty good as well, the older leaves and flowers tend to be bitterer than the younger ones but all are fair game. The roots are an excellent natural source of probiotics which are rich in minerals that you can grind up and use in tea or blend into a fine powder and use in soups and other dishes. The seeds are a natural source of antibiotic and are great for protecting the liver, and can help in fighting infections such as the common cold.

If you google "dandelion kills cancer NCBI" you will see half a dozen scientific studies showing this plant's remarkable power, the study I chose to use is called *"Dandelion root extract affects colorectal cancer proliferation and survival through the activation of multiple death signalling pathways"* by senior research scientist Pamela Ovadje at the Department of Chemistry & Biochemistry at the University of Windsor in Canada. This was the conclusion on Dandelion Root Extract (DRE) in the study.

Our results showed that aqueous dandelion root extract (DRE) efficiently and selectively triggers programmed cell death pathways in in-vitro and in-vivo colorectal cancer models. The results confirmed our hypothesis that the molecular complexity of the DRE extract is responsible for its anti-cancer activity, as it allows the engaging of multiple signalling pathways in cancer cells, including the mitochondria.

Therefore, we can conclude that DRE, as a complex mixture might provide a complementary alternative to currently available chemotherapies. With these results, DRE is approved by Health Canada for Phase I clinical trials in haematological cancers. Their use might prove not only efficacious, but also associated with fewer and less severe side-effects and, thus, improve the quality of life and possibly increase the lifespan of cancer patients.

Uses

All cancer types would benefit from this plant, it would help by cleansing the liver and blood by removing toxins and lactic acid within the body's tissues, it can also aid in removing toxins from the body after conventional treatment. Cancer types that would benefit the most are liver, gallbladder, kidney, colon, leukaemia and any other cancer of the digestive tract or blood. You can even use the stem sap on skin cancers which historically has been used to remove warts and other skin related complaints, the dandelion has also been used to reduce the symptoms and fight off the common cold and pneumonia, great for that COVID 19 governments are fear-mongering over!

So the next time you see one of these plants taking up space in your garden rather than poison it or pull it out of the ground take the leaves and add it to a salad a reap the huge health benefits the humble dandelion has to offer.

Red & White Clover

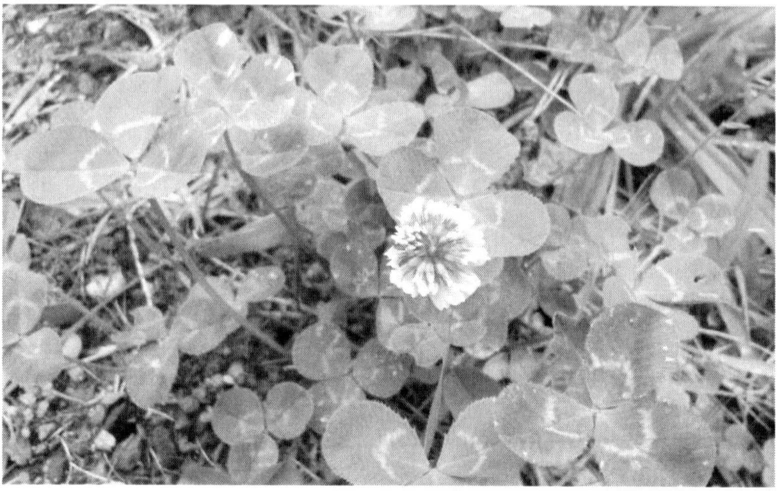

Another fun time favourite of children is to find the elusive four-leaf clover, but more often than not what children find is one of the 900 different varieties of Oxalis that looks like a clover. Believe it or not those little red and white favourites of bees on your lawn are good for cancer and contain high amounts of isoflavones for cancer prevention. Not to be confused with clove, clover contains 4 phytoestrogens which help to regulate hormone balance and protects against estrogen dominance. Clover can help an enlarged prostate, menopause, hot flushes, skin healing, wounds, and psoriasis. It can also alleviate high blood pressure and reduce the risk of blood clots, so it's perfect for people with high cholesterol and those who are at risk of stroke. Clover blossoms are also an expectorant, good for spasmodic coughs, bronchitis, and asthma. The roots of clover can go as far as 128 feet, drawing up all the nutrients and minerals deep in the soil and giving them to you.

Clover is part of the legume family like peas, beans and cashews which most people think is a nut, and historically it has been used to treat cancer, gout, whooping cough and asthma. Although there is limited scientific data to support its effect on cancer it can be used as a cancer preventative because of studies on the high isoflavones which are found in many plants, show the protection against many age-related diseases, loss of cognitive function, cardiovascular disease, osteoporosis, and hormone-dependent cancers like those in the breast, ovaries and thyroid.

Clover is also excellent at fixing nitrogen to the soil and helping other plants grow, so if you see them in your garden or vegetable patch, leave them because they will work wonders for your garden's soil. Do not harvest clover late in the year because it starts to produce poisonous alkaloids, the flower tastes like sweet anise, the leaves and roots are also edible.

Uses:

Any cancer or condition where hormones are the issue, rather than having a direct impact on cancer it can support several aspects of the body. Clover can also keep the blood vessels pliable so you can use it to support all cancer types based on getting oxygen and nutrient-rich blood around the body and to the cancer site to prevent angiogenesis.

Because there are so many varieties of the oxalis family it can be difficult to positively identify clover if it has not flowered. Here are two other members of the oxalis family, the light purple one is called

Arborea and the other is commonly called Wood Sorrel both of which were found in my backyard growing among the clover.

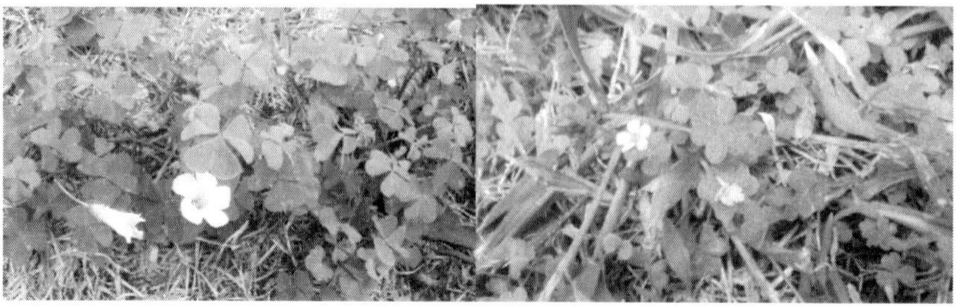

Both of these plants are edible and also have their medicinal uses, they have a very refreshing lemon taste to the leaves and flowers, but because they contain high amounts of oxalic acid they are not to be eaten in large amounts. Perfect for adding to salads and very easy to grow, they can easily be used as a fresh citrus substitute in many dishes. Tea made from these can help with mouth problems like gum infections, they are also a good blood cleanser and great for treating urinary infections, fevers and colds.

WARNING!

Clover does have a toxic lookalike called Crown Vetch, always do your research before using plants and herbs you are unfamiliar with, some are highly toxic! Also, never ferment clover and only eat fresh or dried. It is not recommended for a woman who is pregnant or children, there are many other alternatives.

Yellow Dock

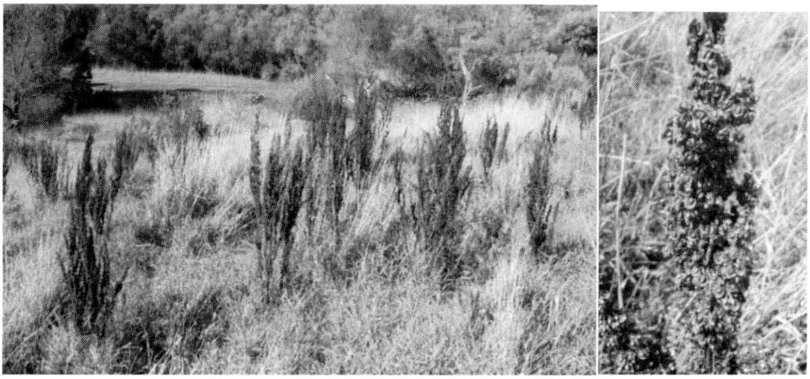

Yellow Dock is also known as Curly Dock or Rumex Crispus, it is found just about everywhere and is another plant considered to be a useless pest to the home garden. This is a body purifying plant! The root contains the most medicinal properties and you should eat the leaves when they are young, it's also a non-irritating laxative for those who have constipation and it can calm the intestines and soothe the intestinal lining, the tea also enhances digestion and improves appetite. The whole plant is useable and yellow dock tea is fairly popular, the seeds turn dark brown, almost black during summer which also has its uses. Yellow dock can be used to detoxify the liver, clean the blood, treat bowel infections, treats peptic ulcers, invigorates the liver and colon with glycosides, great for healing gout, urinary stones, bladder inflammation, soothes respiratory system, helps the body absorb nutrients and purges toxins through the urine. It also contains anthraquinones, which stop ringworm and fungus, it pulls toxins from the blood and raises the red blood cell count and therefore the oxygen supply to the body, great for lymph conditions, inflammation, pain, depression, skin conditions and has been historically used to remove boils, sores, psoriasis and abscesses on the skin. In a study called *"Carbohydrase inhibition and anti-cancerous and free radical scavenging properties along with DNA and protein protection ability of methanolic root extracts of Rumex Crispus"* by researcher Supriya Shiwani at the Department of Medical Biotechnology, College of Biomedical Sciences at Kangwon National University in Korea, said the following in her discussion about Yellow dock (Rumex Crispus).

> *Oxidative DNA damage has been implicated in various degenerative diseases. DNA damage by ROS can initiate carcinogenesis and lead to the pathogenesis of neurodegenerative diseases such as Parkinson's and Alzheimer's disease. Hydroxy radicals are regarded as a DNA damaging agent which can significantly damage the DNA contents of the cells. Though, both 80% methanolic and absolute methanolic RERC was found to be highly potential in DNA protection (HEK 293 cellular DNA) when compared with the positive control. However, 80% methanolic RERC was found to be superior in protecting DNA damage over the other groups.*

Uses

Great for all cancer types and also detoxing from chemotherapy and radiation treatment. Its particularly good for any cancer of the digestive tract, colon, liver, bladder, lymph nodes, lung, skin and blood cancers. Plant around the home in organic soil for a regular harvest of leaves, because the root contains the most medicinal uses it means killing the plant to collect it, if you can't grow enough on your on there is an abundance to harvest in the wild. You can also add the root to normal black tea and add lemon to help overcome the bitter taste.

Chickweed

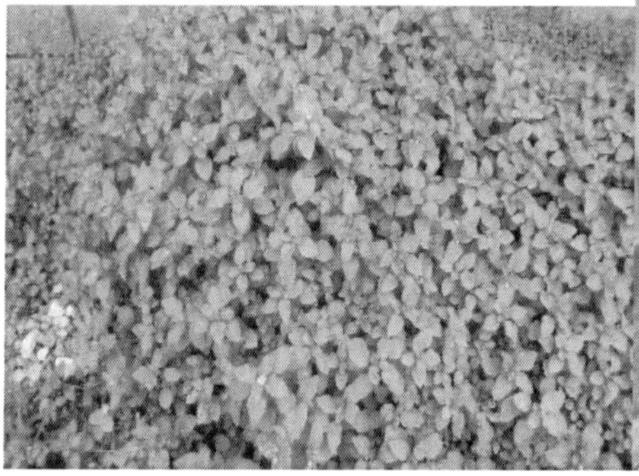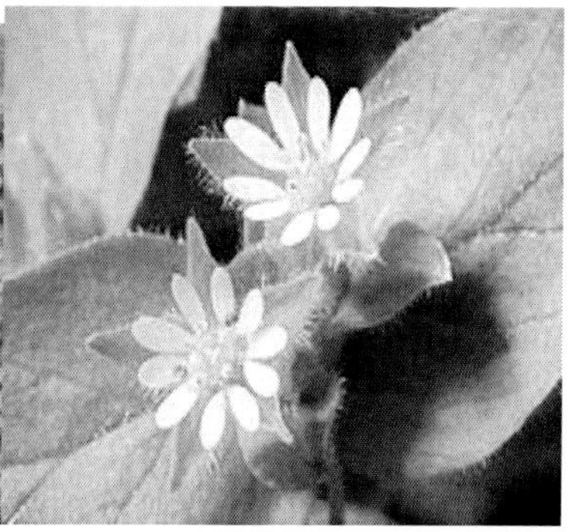

One of the better tasting weeds out there, yet absolute hated by farmers and growers because it has so much vitality it's quite hard to kill. Again another useful plant we are poisoning the shit out of when it could be such a fantastic source of nutrition and health. Chickweed has been used in Chinese medicine for more than 200 years and has many members in its family that share similar characteristics. Chickweed grows all year round, and when using this plant always get the newer leaves, if you go too far down the stem it will be tough and fibrous. Chickweed has anti-inflammatory properties that reduce inflamed lungs, bowels and stomach. It is high in antioxidants and also has an antihistamine which can help to reduce sinus congestion, bronchitis, circulatory problems and the juice is also an antiseptic. It can remove plaque from the arteries, build nerve tissues, regulate the thyroid, can support all cancer types, alkalize the blood, heal ulcers, removes dried mucus from the colon, neutralizes toxins, stimulate lymph glands, laxative properties, kidney issues, rheumatism, high in vitamin C, a complete A & B complex, it has ascorbic acid, beta carotene, calcium, magnesium, niacin, potassium, riboflavin, selenium, thiamine, zinc, copper, and Gamma-linolenic-acid.

The list of what this plant doesn't have would be infinitely shorter and because it grows so quickly cultivating some in a pot has never been so easy.

Uses

Great for all cancer types, particularly useful for cancer of the lungs, bowel, stomach, thyroid, colon, lymph nodes, kidney and all blood cancers. Use in salads or stir fry's or even pick fresh and graze a bit as it is very refreshing to eat and reminds me of crisp snow pea sprouts or watercress in its texture.

WARNING!

Do not take chickweed if you are pregnant! There is also a toxic lookalike called Scarlet Pimpernel which often grows amongst Chickweed so always do your research to make sure you can positively identify what you are about to use. As a rule of thumb, I only pick chickweed when it has flowered so there is no confusion between the two.

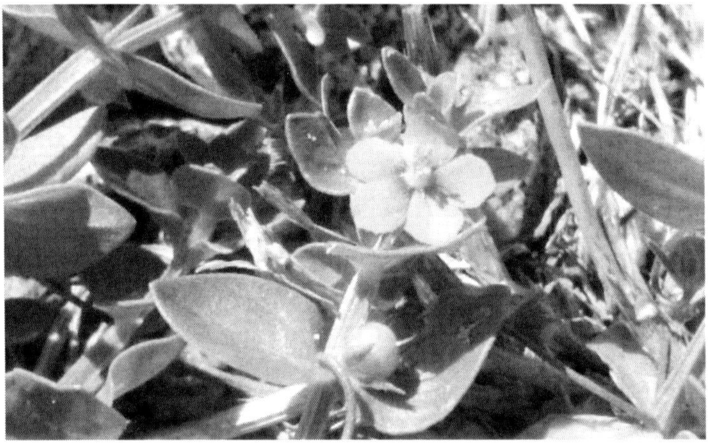

Scarlet Pimpernel (Toxic Lookalike)

Wild Carrot (Queen Anne's Lace)

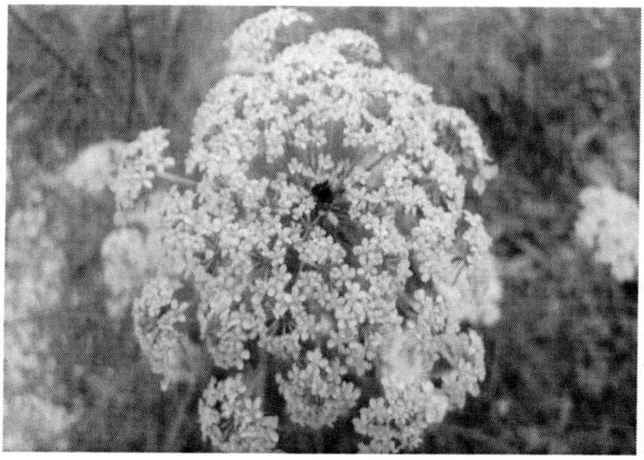

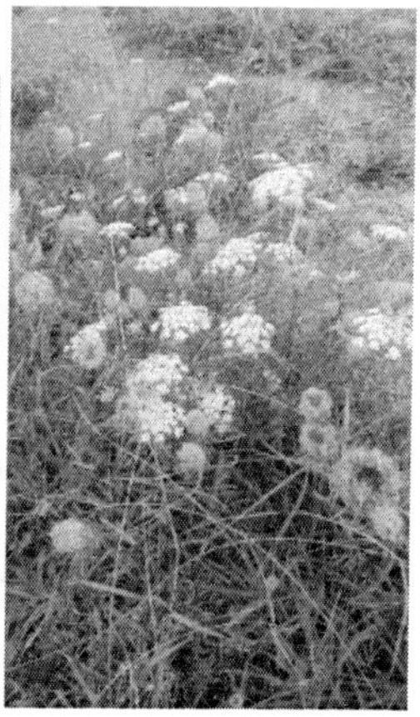

We have all seen this useful plant and its unmistakable white flower, they litter the roadside by the hundreds here in Australia and are found all over the world thanks to international trade.

The reason its called wild carrot is that the roots of first-year plants taste just like a carrot, though they are significantly smaller than a normal carrot after a year the root becomes very tough and is probably not worth digging up. The flowers are used as a diuretic, so it flushes the kidneys of uric acid, the shoots and stems can be eaten raw or steamed and eaten like asparagus. The leaves of wild carrot contain 100 times more vitamin A than an actual carrot and historically it has been used for kidney and bladder issues which is just the beginning of its healing power. Wild Carrot can help with a huge range of health issues including, Alzheimer's, Crohn's disease, Parkinson's, infertility, asthma preventative, all types of cancer, diabetes, leukaemia, HIV symptoms, migraine headache, obesity, stress, PMS, digestive disorders, cystitis, kidney stones and many more.

A study on wild carrots anticancer potential called *"Daucus carota pentane-based fractions arrest the cell cycle and increase apoptosis in MDA-MB-231 breast cancer cells"* by Dr Wassim N Shebaby at the Department of Microbial and Cellular Sciences, Faculty of Health and Medical Sciences at the University of Surrey in the UK concluded the following on wild carrot (Daucus Carota) and its effect on MDA-MB-231.

MDA-MB-231 is an epithelial cell line used in breast cancer studies to determine its effectiveness, to help put this conclusion into context for the unscientifically minded the MAPK/ERK pathway is a chain of proteins in the cell that communicates a signal from a receptor on the surface of the cell to the DNA in the nucleus of the cell. These scientists love their big words but sometimes there is just no substitute for them to explain their results in simple terms because the findings are not simple. Here is what they concluded.

The present study demonstrates that the pentane fraction (F1) and pentane/diethyl ether fraction (F2) have potent anticancer activity against MDA-MB-231 and MCF-7 human breast cancer cells. Both fractions inhibit cell proliferation by inducing cell cycle arrest and apoptosis in MDA-MB-231 cells. This induction of apoptosis is through the inhibition of the ERK pathway. The results suggest that the wild carrot could be considered a potential source for natural anticancer compounds. Future work will focus on isolation and characterization of the tentatively identified major compound and will explore the prospective in vitro and in vivo anticancer capabilities.

Uses

Good for all cancer types and include it in your diet any way you can. Leaves and flowers smell like carrot and can be used in salads, but don't be misled I found it to be quite strong in taste and does not exactly resemble a store-bought carrot as most wild plants don't.

WARNING!

Wild Carrot is part of the umbrella family, and there are many poisonous lookalikes, the one that most closely resembles wild carrot is Poison Hemlock so make sure you know what you are looking for.

I find it ironic that carcinogenic weed killers which may have caused a person's cancer are being used on the very weeds they could be used to prevent it. I would say it's comical and mind-numbingly amusing if it wasn't for the profound impact it is having on people's lives, a true sign of the times and the madness we live in. Today many useful activities that are considered to be exotic interests are some of the most important life skills children should be learning, but instead, children's minds are polluted by society's norms which are getting us nowhere.

Most drugs that your doctor prescribes are derived from plant sources, so why not teach children to develop an appreciation and respect for these wonderful healers before we poison everything and there is nothing left. The chemical Glyphosate which is used to kill these plants is not just ending up in our food but the latest research is showing that it is also responsible for the death of many insect species which are essential to healthy ecosystems.

For fuck sake, do not be another brick in the wall and conform to societies norms because they are nothing to be proud of! We got into this mess by being ignorant, complacent and lazy and whether you choose to accept it or not this mentality has bitten us in the ass big time.

If you are interested in wild plants around the home and want to broaden your botanical knowledge then the book Free Food and Medicine is an absolute must for you to discover new potential cancer healing weeds. On a final note, in case you were wondering, I am in no way shape or form affiliated with Markus Rothkranz or his products, I just loved the simplicity and practical application of the book.

PART VI

CHAPTER 17: THE AGE OF IGNORANCE

I never knew how powerful and widespread ignorance was till this became my life, when we finally got my father home and I was left to take care of him there were many things in this book I did not know. When my father was sent home they gave him anti-inflammatories and some pain killers even though he was in no pain, I said to my mother not to give him the pills from the hospital and that what I had was better. I gave my father high doses of Curcumin found in turmeric and black pepper mixed in with other foods, my most immediate concern was the lesions on his brain; I was giving him close to 30 supplements a day to keep him going because he wasn't eating much. He could barely walk, couldn't talk properly, he was constipated, and his urine looked and smelt very acidic.

After 2 weeks of a controlled diet and all the supplements that I gave him, I woke up one morning around 4 am to the sounds of my mother in her room, my heart sank because I thought he had died in his sleep. I went into my parent's room and to my surprise, he was sitting upright in bed talking to my mother like everything was fine, I couldn't believe the difference, it was as if he was back from the dead or something. Over the next week and a half, he was able to walk with minimal help, ate 3 meals a day, wasn't constipated, was urinating fine and seemed to be making progress. Then around the 4th week he developed a cough with huge amounts of fluid on his lungs, he had caught pneumonia, a common symptom of chemotherapy, this was bad because I knew that if I took him to the doctor they would prescribe him antibiotics which is no better than chemo in the sense that it kills all the good bacteria in the gut, which I had been putting back with probiotics over the last month. Palliative care came around to check on him and said he needs to go to the doctor, so the next day I took him, after being tested by the doctor she said his blood sugar level is normal which was a surprise considering he had secondary cancer in his pancreas, but she said his blood pressure was low and was the reason he looked so flat. Then she said the magic words, he needs an intravenous course of antibiotics to clear the lung infection and needs to be hospitalised, or you can take him home and see how things play out. I admit it took me a while to decide what to do, this was probably the hardest choice I had ever had to make, I knew if he got antibiotics it would be game over, but on the other hand, if I took him home and he died everyone would have blamed me for his death saying that he should have been hospitalised. In the end, I agreed to hospitalize him, it was on the 23rd of September, my 30th birthday. I took him to the hospital and watch doctors pump more shit into his body undoing all the work I had done over the last month. The hospital was so shit that patients had to bring their own tissues when they knew full well that he was coughing up enough fluid to fill 3 shopping bags of tissues a day. After 3 or 4 days he came home and I tried to get him back into the routine of eating healthy, I put his daily food and supplements in front of him and like a child he refused to eat it chucking a tantrum, so I asked him what the problem was? I told him that he had been having this for the last month and all he said to me was, you're poisoning me! Furious by his words, I said "you didn't complain when the doctor was pumping you full of fucking chemo". Fortunately, my mother was home and she had to convince him that what I was giving him wasn't poisoning him and actually helped considering his condition when we brought him home.

He also thought I was starving him, just because I wouldn't give him the things he wanted to eat, my house was a fucking nursery school, and my mind felt like it was breaking in two, how I remained sane till this day I have no idea. After hearing this I sat on my bed and turned on the TV and from out of nowhere I got light headed and this intense fear of dying start to come over me, I quickly realised that I was having some kind of panic or anxiety attack. I tried to center myself and control my breathing and after a minute or so it went away, I thought to myself, these people are fucking kill me! Living with them was unbearable and had it not been for my sense of loyalty and duty to my family I would have taken my chances anywhere else.

It was September the 30th and that night my father kept telling my mother how tired he was, he went to bed that night and around 4 am October the 1st I heard screams coming from my parent's room, I got out of bed so fast I don't even recall getting out of my doona, I ran into the room and he was lying in bed on his side cold as ice, he had died in his sleep sometime during the night. I just remember thinking that at least he wasn't in pain and he went in his sleep which more than anyone could ask for given his condition.

I never got along with my father and over the years I have learned that some parents don't deserve the love of their children. Despite the headaches and the bullshit I still loved him, I just couldn't live with the man, and I'm sure there are many people out there that can relate to this when it comes to their family. My father's death taught me that is ignorance is bliss until something happens, then you are fucked! Turning a blind eye to all of our problems and looking for that magic pill in every medical illness is not the solution, the solution is the evolution of our characters and to learn from our experiences.

We are all ignorant about something, so have no illusions about being the exception to the rule, ignorance is damaging to our way of life and hinders progress. According to James Carse a psychologist and professor at NYU, there are 3 kinds of ignorance where only one is bad and in my opinion unacceptable. There's ordinary ignorance, higher ignorance, and willful ignorance. Ordinary ignorance occurs when you come from a place of not knowing something, to knowing something such as science, history, math and yes, even cancer. The second type is higher ignorance; it is a reverence for the unknown such as God. However, it also allows room for growth because these kinds of people can still be open enough to accept that they don't know something, after all, it is unknown. Finally, the third type is willful ignorance, this occurs when someone knows something and chooses not to believe it because it contradicts what they want reality to be.

We prefer the security of knowing what we think we know and to have evidence's that contradicts or interferes with this understanding is a scenario that is quite terrifying for some people. Challenging people like this with fact on what they think they know and you will often raise a wall that will never be lowered. This is because the person who challenged their beliefs has exercised one of the many freedom's we take for granted. People often believe in the most ridiculous things like Scientology, the tooth fairy, Santa Claus and don't get me started on the Easter Bunny, when was the last time you saw a rabbit lay an egg? Case in point!

Although I respect tradition and have nothing against these fallacies this type of thinking extends into many areas of our lives where people can no longer tell fact from fiction. This includes professionals like doctors and oncologists, they are not immune to this kind of thinking because this is a human problem and they believe what they do because it gives them a type of security. Perhaps adults think this way as a kind of throwback to childhood when their parents provided security and watched over them. But when they became adults that security was gone, so they had to find or create something in its place and this is what their belief system is built on even if it is a lie.

According to Margaret Heffernan entrepreneur, CEO, lecturer and author of five books, "Willful Blindness" is a legal concept where if there is information that you could know, or should know and you manage not too, you have made a conscious choice not to know that information. In Australia legal minds refer to it as ignorance of the law is no excuse, it's an argument that people try to use when they have broken a law, but claim they never knew about the law, otherwise they wouldn't have broken it. I am not entirely unsympathetic to these people concerning the law because we have so many laws in Australia for such stupid shit who can honestly keep up.

In a Ted X speech on Youtube Margaret Heffernan also mentions that willful blindness can be seen everywhere from corporations, governments, large communities and even within the family unit.

We saw it in the banks when they gave people dodgy home loans in the crises leading up to 2008, or the willful blindness in the Catholic church and the decades of child abuse, and also every topic that has been covered in this book.

With so much ignorance in the world, why would anyone think that their oncologist is any less ignorant about cancer causation and treatment than anyone else in any other profession? People see what they want to, they always have, and I don't give a shit what culture you are from, if you are black, white, Asian or fucking rainbow coloured this is a human problem and desperately needs correction.

Willful ignorance and doctors mindsets go back to their formal training and university studies where these doctors are primed and groomed to accept certain information as being useful or factually correct and to disregard the rest. This is why natural or alternative therapies have never found a place in mainstream medicine for diseases like cancer, you have many people out there in the world healing themselves without doctors and their drugs and the vast majority of doctors are not even curious about how they are doing it! This "FACT" alone should be enough to have most people questioning what they are told, yet they blindly continue to give trust that has not been earned. They are not even investigating how these people did it, they are just doing what they were taught, diagnosing problems and fixing them with drugs.

The thing that disturbs me the most is that people seem to be happy that they are oblivious to their surroundings especially here in Australia. The level of ignorance about everything mentioned in this book is unprecedented I would go as far as to say that we have become the country bumkins of the world in terms of these issues. You can see it everywhere if you bother to look, its enslavement by choice! Look at how the police continue to abuse our fundamental human rights, especially during the COVID lockdowns, or because they are just doing what they were told by their superiors who are no wiser than those they instruct. How about our bureaucrats? They have disenfranchised Australian citizens and devastated the Australian economy over the last 40 years by borrowing billions of dollars from a private institution we call the "Reserve Bank of Australia", when we should be taking it from the treasury, that way we don't pay interest on the money we borrow, but instead it's done this way to keep us in debt and dependent on the system we all want to break free from. Its economics 101, if you control the debt you control everything! This is why countries like China will lend money to countries like Africa, because if they default on their debt, then they can take their natural resources as payment. Then these assholes in suits get on television and tell a whole nation what their opinion is when they have no fucking idea what they are talking about and we are supposed to trust, follow or believe these people? This is why voting is a joke, elections are already determined, voting is just a formality to try and give it some legitimacy...

When it comes to cancer and ignorance I never saw a worse case than Peter Hedgemont who was diagnosed by 6 different doctors who all said he had liver cancer, Peter chose not to believe them and he ended up telling his story on the Today Now Show, but tragically Peter died during the interview on national television. I first saw it on Youtube and I see the same level of ignorance everywhere, of course, the last thing I want to do is be insensitive about what happened, nor disrespectful to the departed, but it is a sobering interview to see how he absolutely believes that he does not have cancer and that on national television he proves that his beliefs are absolutely irrelevant to the facts.

To some degree, we have all become like Peter in a way and it is most evident when we blindly trust our experts without ever questioning them or their superiors.

People who are ignorant may be so due to their beliefs which is an interesting subject in itself because belief can be a double edge sword. For example, you could believe that God will heal your cancer because you do not believe in doctors, but in all probability, God won't, you can believe in yourself when accomplishing a specific goal like public speaking or climbing Mount Everest. I do not deny the power of belief and I don't want to say that peoples beliefs don't matter because I have many of my own. Beliefs can give a person the inspiration and confidence to achieve great things, but belief can also deceive a person if it is not realistic, especially when practically applying them to the real world.

Another example would be religion, If you are struggling in life because it conflicts with religious teachings then I would say don't be religious. That doesn't mean you cannot be a spiritual being or a good person, because the truth is that no one on Earth has the answers. I have always said, "religion is the real weapon of mass destruction, not the nuclear bomb, it's not because religious teachings are bad, its because we are too primitive to use them they way they were intended". Think about all of the fucked up shit people have done and continue to do in the name of religion and tell me its not a double edge sword? According to certain religious texts God made man in his image and look at all of the things humanity has done to itself and the life on this planet! Maybe God doesn't make himself known to us because he doesn't want to take credit for the damaged and deranged species we have become? Or maybe he is ashamed of his creation?

Futhermore, if this is how we treat each other and God made us in his image, do you really think this is a God we would want to meet? Ignorance is in every aspect of our lives and is the real evil in humanity!

The placebo effect and belief go hand in hand and many studies show that responses in the body are coming from more than just a sugar pill. Neuroimaging studies have repeatedly shown measurable changes in the neurobiological signaling pathways, and that some studies even show placebos to work just as effective as real drugs. Belief is a powerful tool that when used correctly with supportive treatment can help you overcome many adversities. But conversely, most cancer patients give themselves a nocebo, in the sense that a negative diagnosis can trigger a series of self-destructive psychological thoughts which gives the patient a series of negative physiological responses.

In a short presentation on bias and the brain by Professor Caleb Lack, a clinical psychologist at the University of Central Oklahoma, he talks about how research in the last 15 years has shown that children under the age of 2 are naturally wired to believe in things that are not necessarily there, which contributes to our beliefs in the supernatural later in life. It's interesting that the foundation of what people choose to believe whether it's God, science, ghosts, crystals or whatever, maybe hardwired into our brain probably from birth. It's interesting to see how it can get in the way of thinking logically and critically about a problem, it's almost as if some people cannot distinguish the difference between fact and belief and when they should be used. Instead, people beliefs have become their logic, which is probably why so many people today do such stupid shit.

Willful Ignorance precedes Cognitive Dissonance; Cognitive Dissonance is a term used in psychology when someone has two opposing thoughts at the same time which creates an inconsistency in a person's behaviour, like a person who smokes. They know smoking is bad for them, yet they do it anyway, so logically speaking they shouldn't smoke because it's inconsistent with their thoughts. However, people can add a thought to the mix to try and justify or rationalise the behaviour of smoking by thinking something like an apple a day keeps the doctor away, so smoking probably isn't that bad for me. When it comes to the conventional treatment of cancer this is exactly what you see from your doctor, and it's never been more evident than when the doctor says that the treatment is worse than the disease. Most cancer patients will add a third thought into the mix to justify or rationalise getting conventional treatment, but this kind of thinking by you, your doctor, your friends and family who have all believed that this is how cancer is treated is a lie people tell themselves to reassure that they are making the right choice. Like how smoking is an inconsistent thought, how can you possibly get better from a treatment that makes you worse? There is no logic to this thought what so ever, yet everyone including your doctor seems to accept it.

When people start to change their behaviour to match their thoughts people start waking up to what is going on, it's almost like they were in a zombie apocalypse where everyone around them was stuck in a daydream looking for the butterflies and rainbows in every cup of tea. I have made many people aware of these things over the years and when I do these people come back to me telling me about other crimes and conspiracies like the chemicals in our air, food and water which has contaminated our environment contributing to this toxic feedback loop I was describing earlier. When this happens I usually say "I know exactly what you mean, once you see one you start to see them all, you're starting to see what is really going on and not the narrative you've been told".

One day when this happens to you it may not be because of this book, but someone somewhere is going to say or do something and you will be forced to question your beliefs, and when you wake up and see what's been going on you are going to wonder how the hell you didn't see these things before. I know this because this is how my mother feels, she is completely different to the way she was and she realizes that you cannot take anything today at face value.

When looking at the world with your new eyes a moment of clarity will grab you and you will suddenly experience what we call an epiphany. In this moment of clarity, you will realise that you have to confront the things that you have been taught to ignore your whole life, like the fact that you were living a lie and conforming to a system that does not care about you. It's kind of like the Matrix and you will be forced to make 2 choices, the red pill leads to accepting what has happened and moving on, by leaving what you thought you knew in the past and not dwelling on it so you can now grow and learn from the experience. With your new knowledge, you may want to reach out to friends and family who may be going through a similar ordeal and start to educate them on what's happening around them. Another approach is that you may be pissed off at the fact you have been lied to your whole life and feel the need to become politically active and help spread the word like Jesus of Nazareth preaching peace, love, and equality in the face of this tyranny.

You could do what I did, rather than sitting on all of this knowledge and keeping it to myself I decided to help those in need because I did not want others to suffer unnecessarily as your doctor would have you. You could write a book describing your experiences and try to reach out to as many people as you can, there are millions in this situation right now.

On the other hand, if you choose the blue pill you will be taking a lovely boat ride up that great Egyptian river, DENILE... Rather than waking up, if you prefer to stay in your chemically induced coma and remain in your little dream world then that's entirely your prerogative, but be warned, the world is changing fast and refusing to change with it means you will be left behind. If you or your loved one is on their death bed knowing what is contained in this book and you refused to act, sad to say, but only when it is too late will you know that their death was a too high price to pay for your ignorance. I know what I speak is the truth because that's how my family feels today.

Something that happened only recently to me is something that also deserves attention because of how corrupt it is, I wanted to share it with you to further confirm that I am not full of shit when I speak the fantastic. For this book, I applied for my father's full medical history under a Freedom of Information Request. Here is the reply I was given when I asked for the oncologist's notes, dates and times and other information regarding the 5 years he battled cancer.

easternhealth

Freedom of Information Service
c/- Health Information Services
Maroondah Hospital
PO Box 135, Ringwood East VIC 3135
Tel 03 9871 3170
Fax 03 9871 1653
Email foi@easternhealth.org.au
ABN 68 223 819 017
www.easternhealth.org.au

21 May 2019

Our Ref: B752564 FOI No:23663

Dear JAMES ANDREW

Re: Freedom of Information Request: ALAN ANDREW DOB:14 April 1950

I refer to your request under the Freedom of Information Act 1982 (the FOI Act) for a copy of your late father's Eastern Health medical records.

On 6 May I spoke to you on the phone and you reduced the scope of your request to reports and notes from the oncologist and/or radiologist, in the form of correspondence, and discharge summaries.

You have a right to access those records unless an exemption under the FOI Act Applies.

I have reviewed the medical records and my decision is to release them in part. The part that will not be released is exempt under sections 33(1) and 35(1)(b) of the FOI Act. These exemptions are explained below.

Section 33(1)—the personal privacy exemption—applies to information that relates to the personal affairs of a person (other than your late father) and that would, in the circumstances, be unreasonable to release.

The information considered to be exempt under section 33(1) is information that relates to people who were involved in discussions about your late father's care. Those people are identifiable from that information. It would be unreasonable to release that information because: those people have not consented to its disclosure; that information appears to have been given in confidence; and the release of that information is likely to deter other people from having similar discussions about other patients in the future and this would be detrimental to those patients' care.

Section 35(1)(b) —the exemption relating to material obtained in confidence—applies to information communicated in confidence, which, if disclosed, would impede an agency's ability to obtain similar information in future, and therefore would be contrary (harmful) to the public interest to disclose.

The information considered to be exempt under section 35(1)(b) is information communicated to our service by a persons concerned about your late father's welfare. This information appears to have been given in confidence. If we disclose this type of information, it is likely that other people in the future will not provide similar information in connection with the person they are concerned about. This would be contrary (harmful) to the public interest, and may mean that the person does not get the care they need at that time.

Eastern Health 1300 342 255 *Statewide Services*
Angliss Hospital | Box Hill Hospital | Healesville Hospital and Yarra Valley Health | Maroondah Hospital | Peter James Centre | Wantirna Health | Yarra Ranges Health | Spectrum 03 8833 3050 | Turning Point 03 8413 8413

What they are saying is that without a lawyer subpoenaing the information unedited you cannot access the exact information discussed between your loved ones and what the doctors said because there may be medical negligence.

Here are the sections mentioned in the letter under the FOI so you can read the exact definition.

Section 33(1) - Document Affecting Personal Privacy

A document is an exempt document if its disclosure under this Act would involve the unreasonable disclosure of information relating to the personal affairs of any person (including a deceased person).

The problem I have with this section is that it does not say specifically whose personal information is being protected, family members should have unlimited access to their deceased loved one's information no matter what gets said. However, if it is to do with the oncologist's personal information then why would they tell a patient in the first place if they didn't care about them knowing?

Section 35(1)(b) which says...

The disclosure of the information under this Act would be contrary to the public interest by reason that the disclosure would be reasonably likely to impair the ability of an agency or a Minister to obtain similar information in the future.

So basically they are saying that they will not disclose patient information that will incriminate medical stuff because the public would lose confidence in their ability to do their job. This is no different to someone making an argument that evidence of criminal activity exists but because access to it is being denied by the guilty party no one can make a sound argument for it.

This can only be referred to as the protection of corruption. If you ever plan to do an FOI be prepared for bullshit because they will test your patience and hide behind whatever excuse they can come up, with especially if they are at fault.

I strongly believe that I have fulfilled a deep inner purpose by putting this book together and giving you some of the best that I have to offer. It didn't seem right to know so much information that could help people understand the root cause of their struggle when there are so many people in need. I do not claim to be an expert in anything but then again you don't need to be to tell it how it is. I don't need a maths degree to know that 1 + 1 = 2, nor do I need a degree make it useful in my life. However, for some reason as the mathematical equation grows in complexity and fewer people understand it, society uses this as a means to dismiss what you know because you do not hold a qualification.

I am not one for believing in destiny or fate but I feel as if I have been put on this path to help others in their hour of need. This was made obvious to me when my mother found a letter that I wrote when I was 13 about our dog Sally, which had been long forgotten.

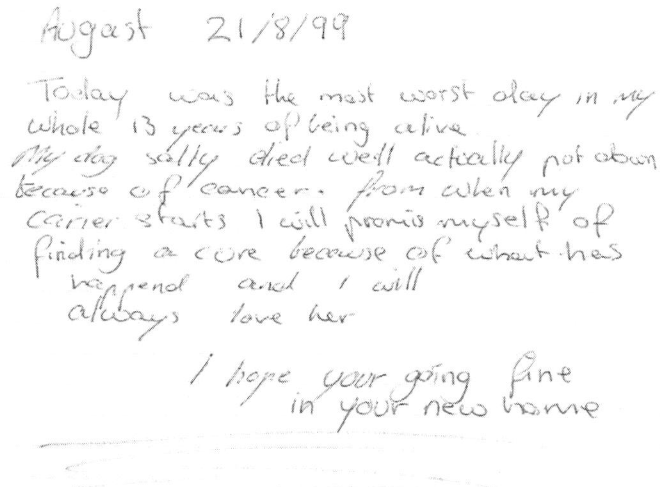
August 21/8/99

Today was the most worst day in my whole 13 years of being alive
My dog sally died well actually not down because of cancer. from when my carier starts I will promis myself of finding a cure because of what has happend and I will always love her

I hope your going fine in your new home

This was a real wake up call for me because it was 21 years ago that I wrote this letter and I had no recollection of writing it until I saw it again. A lot has changed in those 21 years like my shit spelling and grammar, but there are some things that haven't changed like my terrible handwriting and the dream of a 13 year old boy who wanted to right a wrong in a world gone mad. Although I haven't found a "CURE" for cancer I have found many treatments that will help overcome this disease with little to no side effects which I believe is the fulfilment of a promise made to myself a lifetime ago.

If life has side tracked you from what makes you happy then go through those old boxes with a decade's of dust and find who you used to be.

Hopefully by now you understand that there is no one treatment for cancer but dozens, and anything worthy of your time and money sure as shit won't come in a pill, a bottle, or by your oncologist. We need to accept that the troubles we have in this world are something we have done to ourselves, by being complacent and accepting the bullshit that corporations and authority forces upon us, we have given away our power of choice. These entities know that together we are a powerful force to be reckoned with, which is why so many tactics and resources are spent dividing us, together we are strong and what we say goes, but fractured into minority groups like race, gender and religion they pit us against each other sowing hate and distrust.

The power of choice is a hard-won freedom that many people do not exercise and people do not speak out because they feel alone in their struggles when in reality they are not. If we say that we don't want fluoride in our water, chemicals in our food or that vaccination that doesn't work, then tell authority exactly what you think and make a stand. Do not be silent, complacent or obedient if you object to something you never asked for because you are the one that has to drink, eat and get these things, not those who are telling you.

If you want to learn more about what's going on then start looking, ditch the reality TV and your Facebook updates for something that actually brings value to your life. Work hard on making yourself happy and healthy and not just to line some assholes pocket, and if you are an advocate of the message in this book which is to raise awareness on everything that plagues us, then stand against the whole world in defence of your convictions because although many will disagree, you are not wrong. The importance of this message cannot be overstated, with the official doomsday clock moving to 2 mins to midnight in January 2019 many predict that man is headed for the 6th extinction and if we are to avoid this scenario then we must wake up and take action now. Otherwise, the technologies we have created to make our lives easier will become the instruments of our enslavement, and forever keep us slaves to an age of ignorance.

END

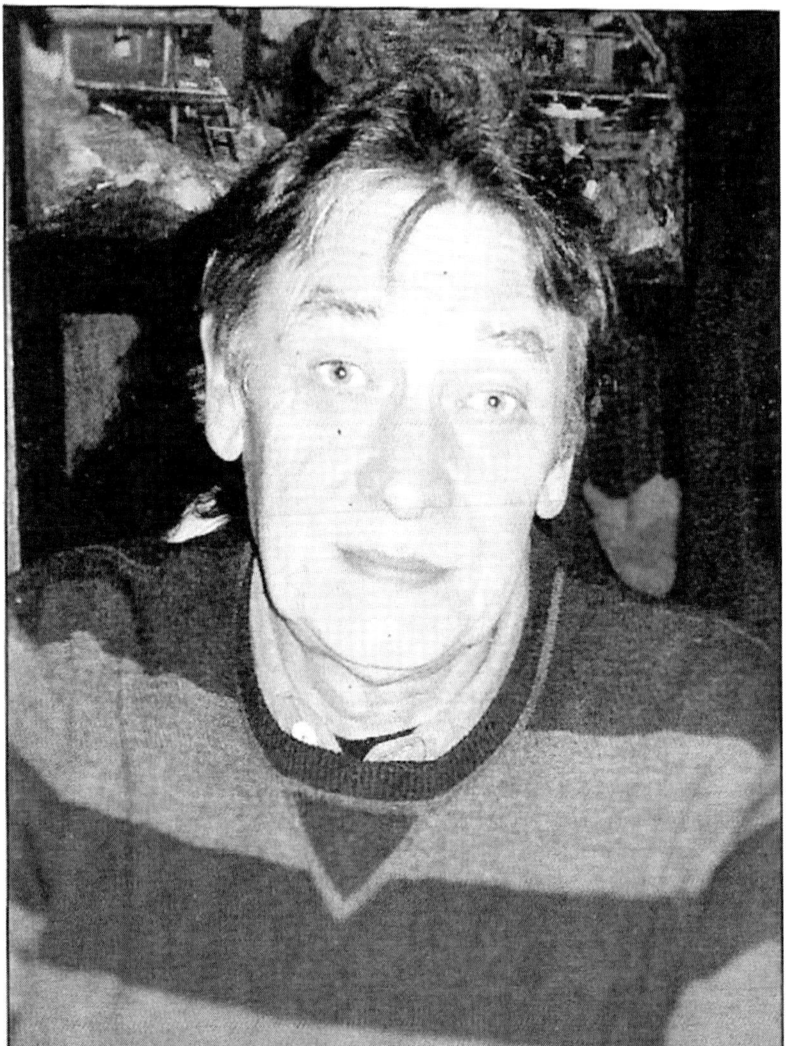

In Loving Memory of Alan Andrew April 14th 1950 – October 1st 2015

Thank You!

☆☆☆☆☆

Dear Customer,

Thank you for joining me on this epic journey! It has been my greatest pleasure to share with you this information and help make a difference in your life.

Please join our FB page at "The Age of Ignorance" to stay up to date with these issues. Also, don't forget to leave a review of this book on Amazon, I cannot stress how important reviews are when it comes to putting this information in front of the people who need it the most.

Best of luck to all of your endeavors,

James Andrew

Cancer Friendly Foods

Vegetables (Organic)

Artichoke, Alfalfa, Alfalfa Sprouts, Avacardo, Argula, Beans (All), Bean Sprouts, Beetroot, Broccoli, Bok Choy, Cabbage (All), Capsicum (All), Cauliflower, Carrots (All), Celery, Celeriac, Collard Greens (All), Corn (All), Chickpeas, Brussel Sprouts, Chives, Chilies (All), Cucumbers (All), Eddoe, Eggplant, Endive, Fennel, Garlic, Ginger, Horseradish, Kale (All), Kelp, Kholrabi, Konjac, kuka, Letils (All), Leek, Lettuce (All), Mustard Greens (All), Nettles, Okra, Onions (All), Parsnips (All), Peas (All), Potato (All), Pumpkins (All), Radish's (All), Radicchio, Rhubarb, rocket, Salsify, Shallots, Silver beet (All), Spinach (All), Tat Soi, Tomato's (All), Turnips, Wasabi, Water Chesnutt, Watercress.

Caution: All Vegetables are fine to eat daily but do not eat any potato variety as a staple it is extremely high in carbohydrates.

Fruits (Organic)

Apples (All), Apricots, Avocado, Bananas, Berries (All), Breadfruit, Cantaloupe, Carambola, Cherimoya, Cherries (all), Citrus (All), Coconut, Custard Apple, Durians, Feijoa, Figs, Grapes (All), Guava (All), Honeydew Melon, Jack Fruit, Java Plum, Kiwi, Kumquat, Logan, Loquat, Lychee, Mango, Nectarine (All), Olives, Papaya, Passion Fruit, Peaches (All), Pears (All), Persimmon, Pitaya, Pineapple, Petagna, Plantain, Plums, Pomegranate, Prickly Pear, Quince, Rhubarb, Rose-Apple, Sapodilla, Soursop, Sugar Apple, Tamarin, Tangerine, Watermelon.

Caution: Fruits are high in sugars so do not eat lots of fruit on a daily basis, the only exception are Berries and Citrus fruits as they are high in nutrients relative to their sugar content.

Mushrooms (Organic)

Any mushroom is fine to eat with cancer but the main ones to focus on are the Reishi Mushroom, Shitake Mushroom and the Maitake Mushroom.

If you have skipped to this section then go to mushrooms so you know how to prepare them.

Nuts & Seeds (Organic)

All nuts are fair game! However, you may want to focus on Almonds, Brazil nuts, Walnuts and Apricot Kernels.

Caution: Do not eat apricot kernels until you have read that section of the book.

Seaweeds (Beach Foraging)

All seaweeds are edible and there are not poisonous edible varieties!

Oils (Organic)

All plant based cooking oils are fine to cook with. You will get the most benefits out of Extra Virgin olive oil, Clove Oil, Coconut oil, Hemp oil & Frankincense oil.

Caution: Do not use Canola or Vegetable oil, they are heavily GMO.

Herbs & Spices (Organic)

The list of useable herbs and spices are endless, that said all are fine to use. However, you will want to make a select few a regular staple in your diet and they are the following:

All Spice, Basil, Black Pepper, Caraway, Cardamom, Cinnamon, Clove, Coriander, Cumin, Dill, Garlic, Ginger, Ginseng, Pink Himalayan Salt, Rosemary, Saffron, Turmeric & Tyme.

Supplements & Probiotics

There are tons of supplements out their today so as rule of thumb you are after Organic/Plant based supplements nothing synthetic like most vitamin C tablets. So here is a short list of supplements every cancer patient should be taking to plug the gaps in their diet.

Probiotic

Inner health plus – You are looking for a broad spectrum probiotic, not Yakult which is high in sugar or 10 billion of just one variety, diversity is key.

Supplements

Multivitamin – You will need a good quality multivitamin

Resveratrol – There are many benefits to resveratrol including some anti-cancer effects, improves blood work, good for brain and extension of life.

Curcumin – Is a potent anti-inflammatory, has anti-cancer benefits, is immune boosting, helps with arthritis pain, eases depression and whole bunch more.

Vitamin D – These are not as good as natural sunlight be if you have had any bloodwork done and you are low in something, chances are your vitamin D is down and everything else as well.

These 5 supplements are the bare bones of what you should be taking, there are many more and there is a ton of research out there on the effects all of these can have on cancer

If you have skipped to this section to see what you can eat immediately then do not deviate from this list. While recovering do not eat any meat or dairy until you understand why these foods are to be avoided, to put this list into context the book must be read in its entirety.

I sincerely hope that this aids in your endeavors...

Detoxification Schedule

Week	Cleanse Type	Ingredients/Actions
1	Skin Detox (Ongoing)	Baths not Showers Add 2 cups of Sea Salt and 2 cups of Bicarb Soda. Have as hot as you can stand & stay in for at least 45min until cool. Do not add more hot water.
2	Colon Cleanse	Buy or distil 2 litres of water........ Buy raw non-pasteurised organic apple cider vinegar, organic lemons and aloe Vera juice. Add 4 tablespoons of apple cider vinegar, add the juice of 1 lemon & 2 tablespoons of Aloe Vera juice
3	Bacteria in the Gut (Ongoing)	Use a broad spectrum probiotic such as inner health plus and take on an empty stomach.
4	Liver & Gallbladder Cleanse (Ongoing)	Buy malic acid tables to soften liver stones and take daily. Then make a tea or tonic from dandelion root, milk thistle and lemon and drink daily. This cleanse should be on going, it will not take a week to remove liver stones they are difficult to remove.
5	Parasite Cleanse	Go to your chemist and ask them for their best over the counter parasite flush. It's that easy!

6	Chemical & Heavy Metal Cleanse (At least 2 weeks)	Get your hands on some food grade bentonite clay form a health food store. Mix bentonite clay, activated charcoal and a cup of organic coriander. Do not use a metallic spoon to mix If you feel any symptoms such as headaches after

Note: Some of these cleanses will be ongoing and others will take about a week. It's important to note that this is not an overnight fix and that this schedule should be repeated from week 2 once you have completed week 6.

References...

A. Alfred Taubman Medical Research Institute. (Mar 12, 2013). *Cancer Stem Cells - Max Wicha, M.D.* [Video file]. Retrieved from https://www.youtube.com/watch?v=AG22BEXscQE

ABC Evening News 2013-03-21. (March 21st 2013). *Television Vanderbilt News Archive.* Retrieved from https://tvnews.vanderbilt.edu/programs/1040717

Adithya Cattamanchi, MD. (Thu 15 November 2018). *What to know about lung cancer.* Retrieved from https://www.medicalnewstoday.com/articles/323701.php

A Eramo, T L Haas & R De Maria. Department of Hematology, Oncology and Molecular Medicine, Istituto Superiore di Sanità, Viale Regina Elena 299, Rome, Italy. Lung cancer stem cells: tools and targets to fight lung cancer. (August 2010). *NCBI Pub Med.* Retrieved from https://www.ncbi.nlm.nih.gov/pubmed/20531299

Akimoto M., Iizuka M., Kanematsu R., Yoshida M., Takenaga K. Anticancer effect of ginger extract against pancreatic cancer cells mainly through reactive oxygen species-mediated autotic cell death. *PLoS ONE,* 10 (5), art. no. e0126605. (2015). Retrieved from https://journals.plos.org/plosone/article/metrics?id=10.1371/journal.pone.0126605#citedHeader

Alexandra Sims. Breast cancer isn't sexy. Woman shares post-radiation images to show reality of disease. (October 25th

2015). *Independent.* Retrieved from https://www.independent.co.uk/life-style/health-and-families/health-news/breast-cancer-isn-t-sexy-woman-shares-post-radiation-images-to-show-reality-of-disease-a6709516.html

Alexis Duclos. Agent Orange Victims in Vietnam. (December 2004). *Wikimedia Commons.* Retrieved from https://commons.wikimedia.org/w/index.php?curid=3431528

Alieva, M., van Rheenen, J., & Broekman, M. (2018). Potential impact of invasive surgical procedures on primary tumor growth and metastasis. *Clinical & experimental metastasis, 35*(4), 319–331. doi:10.1007/s10585-018-9896-8

American Cancer Society. How does chemotherapy affect the risk of second cancers. (n.d). *American Cancer Society.* Retrieved from https://www.cancer.org/treatment/treatments-and-side-effects/physical-side-effects/second-cancers-in-adults/chemotherapy.html

Ammonia (NH3): Uses & Benefits. (n.d*). Studious Guy.* Retrieved from https://studiousguy.com/ammonia-nh3-uses-benefits/

Ammonium Hydroxide ACS. (21/11/2016). *Labchem.* Retrieved from http://www.labchem.com/tools/msds/msds/LC11050.pdf

An Alternative Theory on Cancer. (June 27, 2007). *Medical X Press.* Retrieved from https://medicalxpress.com/news/2007-06-alternative-theory-cancer.html

Ancient Code. (n.d). *Ancient Code.* Retrieved from https://www.ancient-code.com/ica-stones-20-fascinating-rare-images-controversial-stones/

Andrea Billups. How much revenue do vaccines generate. (June 27th 2015). *Newsmax Independent American.* Retrieved from https://www.newsmax.com/FastFeatures/vaccines-revenue/2015/06/27/id/652549/

Angus Thompson. Man claims he was fined $200 for emptying water bottle. (February 24, 2012). *News.com.au.* Retrieved from https://www.news.com.au/national/man-claims-he-was-fined-200-for-emptying-water-bottle/news-story/9eb8664e6ecb19a5eb4fcb196fee53b0

Anna Scanlon. These 7 Turmeric Brands are Being Recalled Due to Lead Contamination. (August 12th 2016). *Natural Society.* Retrieved from http://naturalsociety.com/turmeric-recalled-due-to-high-lead-levels-5546/

Ann Hibner Koblitz. Agent Orange and Abortion in Vietnam. (April 14th 2014). *ahkoblitz~ Sex, Abortion, and Contraception.* Retrieved from https://ahkoblitz.wordpress.com/2014/04/14/agent-orange-and-abortion-in-vietnam/

Aravind A, Dhanya RS, Narayan A, Sam G, Adarsh VJ, Kiran M. Effect of fluoridated water on intelligence in 10-12-year-old school children. (Suppl 3):S237-S242. (December 2016). *NCBI PubMed.* Retrieved from https://www.ncbi.nlm.nih.gov/pubmed/28217543

Autism. (2018). *First Immune Biotech.* Retrieved from https://gcmaf.se/autism/

Bharat B. Aggarwal. *Nature Reviews Immunology* 3, 745–756. Signalling pathways of the TNF superfamily: A double-edged sword. (September 1st 2003). *Nature Review Immunology.* Retrieved from https://www.nature.com/articles/nri1184

Bill Otinger. (Oct 26, 2009). *Hitler & fluoride added high dose to water at concentration camps keep people like walking dead.* [Video file]. Retrieved from https://www.youtube.com/watch?v=3dZPOJ4p1DM

Binder, M., Roberts, C., Spencer, N., Antoine, D., & Cartwright, C. (2014). On the antiquity of cancer: evidence for metastatic carcinoma in a young man from ancient Nubia (c. 1200 BC). *PloS one, 9*(3), e90924. doi:10.1371/journal.pone.0090924

BioDigital, Inc. (Oct 14, 2008). *3D Medical Animation - What is Cancer?.* [Video File]. Retrieved from https://www.youtube.com/watch?v=LEpTTolebqo

Bitesize. Radioactive emissions. (n.d). *BBC.* Retrieved from https://www.bbc.com/bitesize/guides/z2r7ng8/revision/2

Blagosklonny MV. Cancer Center, Ordway Research Institute, Albany, New York 12208, USA: Molecular theory of cancer. (June 5th 2005). *NCBI PubMed.* Retrieved from https://www.ncbi.nlm.nih.gov/pubmed/15970666

Bozeman Science. (Apr 12, 2014). *What is Cancer?.* [Video File]. Retrieved from https://www.youtube.com/watch?v=UopUxkeC4Ls

Breast cancer conference. Philippa D Darbre – Philippa D Darbre | Breast Cancer 2015 | Conferenceseries LLC. (Apr 23, 2016). *Youtube.* Retrieved from https://www.youtube.com/watch?v=5FFaDoAiqo0

Buehring GC[1], DeLaney A[2], Shen H[3], Chu DL[4], Razavian N[5], Schwartz DA[6,7], Demkovich ZR[8], Bates MN[3]. School of Public Health, University of California, 16 Barker Hall, Berkeley, CA, 94720-7354, USA .Bovine Leukaemia virus discovered in human blood. (April 02, 2019). *NCBI PubMed.* Retrieved from https://www.ncbi.nlm.nih.gov/pubmed/30940091

Cancer Net Editorial Board. Side Effects of Radiation Therapy. (December 2016). *Cancer.net.* Retrieved from https://www.cancer.net/navigating-cancer-care/how-cancer-treated/radiation-therapy/side-effects-radiation-therapy

Cancer risk in 680,000 people exposed to computed tomography scans in childhood or adolescence: data linkage study of 11 million Australians. BMJ 2013;346:f2360. (May 21st 2013). Retrieved from https://www.bmj.com/content/346/bmj.f2360

Cancer Treatment Centers of America - CTCA. (Oct 31, 2013). *What is cancer? | What causes cancer and how is it treated.* [Video file]. Retrieved from https://www.youtube.com/watch?v=SGaQ0WwZ_0I

Causes of Breast Cancer. (n.d). *National Breast Cancer Foundation.* Retrieved from https://www.nationalbreastcancer.org/causes-of-breast-cancer

Charles Q. Choi. Can Sugar Make You Stupid? "High Concern" in Wake of Rat Study. (May 23rd 2012). *National Geographic News.* Retrieved from https://news.nationalgeographic.com/news/2012/05/120522-sugar-stupid-rats-high-fructose-corn-syrup-health-science/

Child Health Safety. Vaccines did not save us – 2 centuries of official statistics. (n.d). *Childhealthsafety.com.* Retrieved from https://childhealthsafety.wordpress.com/graphs/

Chris Ariens. Remembering David Aponte. (June 29th 2013). *ABC People TV Newser.* Retrieved from https://www.adweek.com/tvnewser/remembering-david-aponte/187402/

Chris Wark. The Top 10 Anti-Cancer Vegetables. (n.d). *Chris Beat Cancer.* Retrieved from https://www.chrisbeatcancer.com/top-10-anti-cancer-vegetables/

Coleen Codekas & Joel Schwartz. Chickweed. (March 18th, 2019). *Grow, forage, cook, ferment.* Retrieved from https://www.growforagecookferment.com/foraging-for-chickweed/

Connor J[1]. Department of Preventive and Social Medicine, University of Otago, New Zealand. Alcohol consumption as a cause of cancer. (July 21st 2016). *NCBI PubMed.* Retrieved from https://www.ncbi.nlm.nih.gov/pubmed/27442501

Coombs NJ[1], Taylor R, Wilcken N, Fiorica J, Boyages J. New South Wales Breast Cancer Institute, University of Sydney, Westmead Hospital, Westmead, New South Wales, Australia. Hormone replacement therapy and breast cancer risk in California. (Nov-Dec 2005). *NCBI PubMed.* Retrieved from https://www.ncbi.nlm.nih.gov/pubmed/16297085

CSI. The History of Ginseng. (n.d). *CSI Ginseng Products Inc.* Retrieved from http://www.csiginseng.com/history.htm

Cytoluminator. (January 20th 2018). *An Alternative theory on cancer.* Retrieved from http://cancer.cytoluminator.com/alternative-cancer-theory.html

David Freeman. 12 Health Risks of Chronic Heavy Drinking. (n.d). *WebMD.* Retrieved from https://www.webmd.com/mental-health/addiction/features/12-health-risks-of-chronic-heavy-drinking#1

Dena Schmidt. New study: Eating organic food lowers cancer risk. (October 30, 2018). *Natural Health 365.* Retrieved from https://www.naturalhealth365.com/organic-food-news-2752.html

Dórea J. G. (2015). Exposure to mercury and aluminum in early life: developmental vulnerability as a modifying factor in neurologic and immunologic effects. *International journal of environmental research and public health, 12*(2), 1295–1313. doi:10.3390/ijerph120201295

Dr Ananya Mandal, MD, Reviewed by Sally Robertson B.Sc. Gene Therapy History. (n.d). *News Medical Life Sciences.* Retrieved from https://www.news-medical.net/health/Gene-Therapy-History.aspx

Dr. Edward Group. (n.d). *7-Day Oxygen Colon Cleanse Instructions.* Retrieved from https://www.globalhealingcenter.com/cleansing/7-day-oxygen-colon-cleanse

Dr. Edward Group DC, NP, DACBN, DCBCN, DABFM. Why I'm Concerned About the Dangers of Aluminum. (July 17, 2013). *Global Healing Centre.* Retrieved from https://www.globalhealingcenter.com/natural-health/concerned-about-aluminum-dangers/

Dr. Edward Group DC, NP, DACBN, DCBCN, DABFM. The Hidden Formaldehyde in Everyday Products. (October 21, 2015). *Global healing centre.* Retrieved from https://www.globalhealingcenter.com/natural-health/formaldehyde/

Dr. Josh Axe. DC, DMN, CNS. Glutathione: Top 9 Foods & Supplements to Boost. (August 31, 2018). *Dr Axe Food is*

Medicine. Retrieved from https://draxe.com/glutathione/

Dr. Josh Axe, DC, DMN, CNS. Reishi Mushroom: Fight Cancer, Boost Immunity & Improve Liver Detox. (September 11, 2018). *Dr. Axe food is medicine.* Retrieved from https://draxe.com/reishi-mushroom/

Dr. Josh Axe, DC, DMN, CNS. Raw Milk Benefits Skin, Allergies and Immunity. (March 13, 2014). *Dr. Axe – Food is Medicine.* Retrieved from https://draxe.com/raw-milk-benefits/

Dr. Josh Axe. (Apr 21, 2015.) *Benefits of Bentonite Clay.* [Video file]. Retrieved from https://www.youtube.com/watch?v=D_lhVbFFaYs

Dr. Mecola and Dr. Shade Ph.D. The three pillars of heavy metal detoxification. (June 19th, 2016. *Mercola take control of your health.* Retrieved from https://articles.mercola.com/sites/articles/archive/2016/06/19/heavy-metal-detoxification.aspx

Dr Poonam Gusain and Vir Singh, GB Pant University of Agriculture & Technology Pantnagar: Interesting Fact Notes About Deadly Poisonous Plants. (December 28th 2015). *Scientific India.* Retrieved from http://www.scind.org/229/Science/interesting-fact-notes-about-deadly-poisonous-plants.html

Edelson, S. SciBX. Figure 1: Ammonia as a stress signal in cancer. (May 13th 2010). *Science Business Exchange.* Retrieved from https://www.nature.com/scibx/journal/v3/n19/fig_tab/scibx.2010.578_F1.html

Ekos TV. The Fluoride Conspiracy. (Aug. 25, 2006). *Information Liberation.* Retrieved from http://www.informationliberation.com/?id=14949

Elizabeth Pennisi. Monkey Virus DNA Found in Rare Human Cancers. Vol. 275, Issue 5301, pp. 748-749 DOI: 10.1126/science.275.5301.748 (February 7th 1997). *ScienceMag.com.* Retrieved from https://science.sciencemag.org/content/275/5301/748.long

Emilio Labrador from Davie (South Florida). Agent Orange Victims. (May 1, 2015). *Wikimedia commons.* Retrieved from https://commons.wikimedia.org/w/index.php?curid=39888266

Erin Elizabeth. (Aug 12, 2015). *Health Nut News.* Retrieved from https://www.healthnutnews.com/video-dr-jeffrey-bradstreets-family-breaks-silence-for-the-first-time-since-his-tragic-death/

Esoteric Extraterrestrial. (Nov 23, 2015). *The greater good think you know everything about vaccines, think again.* [Video file]. Retrieved from https://www.youtube.com/watch?v=DqOzvYwcLpE

Evidence mounts for link between opioids and cancer growth. (March 21, 2012). *At the Forefront – U Chicago Medicine.* Retrieved from https://www.uchicagomedicine.org/forefront/news/201

2/march/evidence-mounts-for-link-between-opioids-and-cancer-growth

Facts and figures. (n.d). *Cancer Council Australia.* Retrieved from https://www.cancer.org.au/about-cancer/what-is-cancer/facts-and-figures.html

Fernanda Martini, Alfredo Corallini, Veronica Balatti, Silvia Sabbioni, Cecilia Pancaldi and Mauro Tognon. Infectious Agents and Cancer - Simian virus 40 in humans. (July 9, 2007, Volume 2, Number 1, Page 1). *BMC Part of Springer Nature.* Retrieved from https://infectagentscancer.biomedcentral.com/articles/10.1186/1750-9378-2-13

Fiona Macrae. Cancer 'is purely man-made' say scientists after finding almost no trace of disease in Egyptian mummies. (15 October 2010). *The Daily Mail Australia.* Retrieved from https://www.dailymail.co.uk/sciencetech/article-1320507/Cancer-purely-man-say-scientists-finding-trace-disease-Egyptian-mummies.html

Fleur Hupston. Top foods that chelate the body of heavy metals. (January 14th, 2013). *Natural news.* Retrieved from https://www.naturalnews.com/038670_heavy_metals_chelation_foods.html

FluorideAction. (Mar 9, 2011). *The History of Fluoride from the 'Fluoride Deception.* [Video file]. Retrieved from https://www.youtube.com/watch?v=gAg8saQWhiI

George Chernilevsky. Human Gallstones all removed in one patient. Grid Scale 1mm. (October 26, 2015). *Wikipedia*

Commons. Retrieved from https://commons.wikimedia.org/wiki/File:Human_gallstones_2015_G1.jpg

Gertrude C. Buehring, HuaMin Shen, Daniel A. Schwartz, James S. Lawson. Bovine leukemia virus linked to breast cancer in Australian women and identified before breast cancer development. (June 22, 2017). *PLOS ONE.* Retrieved from https://journals.plos.org/plosone/article/authors?id=10.1371/journal.pone.0179367

Harvard Men's Health Watch. Selenium and Prostate cancer. (March, 2007). *Harvard Health Publishing – Harvard Medical School.* Retrieved from https://www.health.harvard.edu/newsletter_article/selenium-and-prostate-cancer

Healing Power Hour. (Aug 29, 2011). *The Health Benefits of Ginger.* [Video file]. Retrieved from https://www.youtube.com/watch?v=6LN2QDaQr38

Heather McClees. This is how dairy affects your hormones. Get ready to ditch dairy today. (January 2019). *One Green Planet.* Retrieved from https://www.onegreenplanet.org/natural-health/how-dairy-affects-your-hormones/

Hewitt M, Weiner SL, Simone JV. Institute of Medicine (US) and National Research Council (US) National Cancer Policy Board. Childhood Cancer Survivorship: Improving Care and Quality of Life. Washington (DC): National Academies Press US. (2003). *NCBI Bookshelf.* Retrieved from https://www.ncbi.nlm.nih.gov/books/NBK221740/

iHealthTube.com. (Aug 14, 2012). *Fluoride is dangerous and doesn't help teeth!.* [Video file]. Retrieved from https://www.youtube.com/watch?v=GlUYKEycUxA

Immunocentre. (10th February 2018). *GcMAF.* Retrieved from https://www.immunocentre.eu The Human Genome Project. *(October 1, 2015). National Human Genome Research Institute.* Retrieved from https://www.genome.gov/10001772/all-about-the--human-genome-project-hgp/

Ingrid Moen, Charlotte Jevne[†],Jian Wang, Karl-Henning Kalland, Martha Chekenya, Lars A Akslen, Linda Sleire, Per Ø Enger, Rolf K Reed, Anne M Øyan and Linda EB Stuhr. Gene expression in tumor cells and stroma in dsRed 4T1 tumors in eGFP-expressing mice with and without enhanced oxygenation. (January 17, 2012). *BMC Part of Springer Nature.* Retrieved from https://bmccancer.biomedcentral.com/articles/10.1186/1471-2407-12-21

Jack D. Thrasher & Kaye H. Kilburn. Embryo Toxicity and Teratogenicity of Formaldehyde, Archives of Environmental Health. Pages 300-311, DOI: 10.1080/00039890109604460. (April, 1 2001). *An International Journal.* Retrieved from http://www.tandfonline.com/doi/abs/10.1080/00039890109604460

Jay W. Marks, MD. *(1/26/2018). Colon Polyps Symptoms, Causes, Types, Treatment and Prevention.* Retrieved from https://www.medicinenet.com/colon_polyps/article.htm

Jdfly. Topic: why is no one talking about Radionecrosis of the breast?. (September 1st 2016). *Breast Cancer. Org Community.* Retrieved from https://community.breastcancer.org/forum/70/topics/847635?page=2

Joe Graedon. Do prescription drugs cause cancer. (October 20th 2008). *The people's pharmacy.* Retrieved from https://www.peoplespharmacy.com/2008/10/20/do-prescription-1/

John Beard, D.SC with a foreword by Nicholas J, Gonzalez, M.D. The enzyme treatment of cancer and its scientific basis. (n.d). *The New Spring Press.* Retrieved from https://www.newspringpress.com/beard.html

John Hall. Why scented candles could cause cancer. (January 16, 2016). *The Telegraph.* Retrieved from https://www.telegraph.co.uk/news/health/news/12103003/Why-scented-candles-could-cause-cancer.html

Johnson & Johnson ordered to pay $4.7bn over talc cancer claims. (July 2018). *The Guardian Australian Edition.* Retrieved from https://www.theguardian.com/business/2018/jul/13/johnson-johnson-ordered-to-pay-47bn-in-talc-powder-claim

Joseph C DiNardo MS. Craig A Downs PhD. Dermatological and environmental toxicological impact of the sunscreen ingredient oxybenzone/benzone/benzophenone-3.

(October 31, 2017). *NCBI PubMed).* Retrieved from https://www.ncbi.nlm.nih.gov/pubmed/29086472

Judd Handler. How the rest of the world brushes its teeth. (October 6th 2015). *MNN.com.* Retrieved from https://www.mnn.com/health/fitness-well-being/stories/how-the-rest-of-the-world-brushes-their-teeth

Kaldari. Common Chickweed (Stellaria Media) in Nashville, Tennessee. Each Flower is approximately 5 mm across. Focus stacked from two images. (28 March 2010). *Wikipedia Commons.* Retrieved from https://commons.wikimedia.org/wiki/File:Kaldari_Stellaria_media_01.jpg

Kanika Khara. The Amazing uses of Lead that make it a versatile metal. (Apr 30, 2018). *Sciencestruck.* Retrieved from https://sciencestruck.com/uses-of-lead

Kate Arney. Claims that cancer is only a 'modern, man-made disease' are false and misleading. (October 4th 2010). *Cancer research UK.* Retrieved from https://scienceblog.cancerresearchuk.org/2010/10/14/claims-that-cancer-is-only-a-%E2%80%98modern-man-made-disease%E2%80%99-are-false-and-misleading/

Kate Daniels. Essiac tea for detox and cancer treatment. (n.d). *A.R.A.I.* Retrieved from http://aidshivawareness.org/essiac-tea-for-detox-and-cancer-treatment/

Keele University. (Dec 8, 2016). *The Age of Aluminium (Die Akte Aluminium).* [Video file]. Retrieved from

https://www.youtube.com/watch?v=5F0u54gs0iU
Lifestyle Medicine. (Oct 5, 2014). *All The Health Benefits of Probiotics in 90*

Key Cancer Statistics. (n.d). *World Health Organization.* Retrieved from https://www.who.int/cancer/resources/keyfacts/en/*Sec onds.* [Video file]. Retrieved from https://www.youtube.com/watch?v=mlWduhHH3LQ

Laforest L, Luce D, Goldberg P, *et al.* Laryngeal and Hypopharyngeal cancers and occupational exposure to formaldehyde and various dusts: A case-control study in France. Volume 57, Issue 11, 2000;57:767-773. (n.d). *BMJ Journals, Occupational and Environmental Medicine.* Retrieved from. https://oem.bmj.com/content/57/11/767.short

Larry Cook. The dangers of vaccines and vaccinations. (n.d). *Stop mandatory vaccination.* Retrieved from http://www.stopmandatoryvaccination.com/vaccine-dangers/

Lead Production & Statistics. (n.d). *International Lead Association.* Retrieved from https://www.ila-lead.org/lead-facts/lead-production--statistics

Learn the Risks.org. Brandy Vaughn. (n.d.). *Death from common infectious diseases Declined by 90% before vaccines were introduced.* Retrieved from https://learntherisk.org/diseases/

Lecia Bushak. From Ancient Tumors To Today's Breakthroughs: A Brief History Of Cancer. (Jun 25, 2015). *Medical Daily.* Retrieved from https://www.medicaldaily.com/ancient-tumors-todays-breakthroughs-brief-history-cancer-339818

Life Strength FC. (Oct 21, 2016). *Vaxxed: from Cover-Up to Catastrophe.* [Video file]. https://www.youtube.com/watch?v=u0Cy3xi62m0

Lis Da MD. 12 Health Benefits of Yellow Dock (No.5 For Deadly Diseases). (April 23rd, 2016). *Dr. Health benefits.* Retrieved from https://drhealthbenefits.com/herbal/leaves/the-health-benefits-of-yellow-dock

Love thy neighbour as thyself. (Feb 25, 2016). *Vaccine Nation (Documentary).* [Video file]. Retrieved from https://www.youtube.com/watch?v=bLk641P8CE4

Ludwig DS, Willett WC. Three Daily Servings of Reduced-Fat Milk: An Evidence-Based Recommendation? *JAMA Pediatr.* 2013;167(9):788–789. doi:10.1001/jamapediatrics.2013.2408. (September 2013). *Jama Network- Jama Paediatrics.* Retrieved from https://jamanetwork.com/journals/jamapediatrics/article-abstract/1704826

Lynne Eldridge, MD. Managing Effects of Radiation Therapy. (January 14, 2019). *Very well Health.* Retrieved from https://www.verywellhealth.com/managing-effects-of-radiation-therapy-2249335

Maitake. For patients and care givers. (November 8, 2018). *Memorial Sloan Kettering cancer clinic.* Retrieved from https://www.mskcc.org/cancer-care/integrative-medicine/herbs/maitake

Majerovich, J. A., Canty, A., & Miedema, B. (2010). Chronic vulvar irritation: could toilet paper be the culprit?. *Canadian family physician Medecin de famille canadien, 56*(4), 350–352.

Mark P Brady, MS, PA-C. Re-emergence of 5 vaccine preventable diseases. (May 14th 2015). *MedScape.* Retrieved from https://reference.medscape.com/features/slideshow/vaccine-preventable-diseases

Mark Strauss. Earliest Human Cancer Found in 1.7-Million-Year-Old Bone. (July 28th 2016). *National Geographic.* Retrieved from https://news.nationalgeographic.com/2016/07/oldest-human-cancer-disease-origins-tumor-fossil-science/

MarshallU. (Sep 1, 2011). *Marshall University: Walnuts and Cancer Research.* [Video File]. Retrieved from https://www.youtube.com/watch?v=r5dDqCS_NiA

Martha Whitney. Ginger. (n.d). *Dr Christophers Herbal Legacy.* Retrieved from http://www.herballegacy.com/Whitney_History.html

Matsui T[1], Matsukawa Y, Sakai T, Nakamura K, Aoike A, Kawai K. Effect of ammonia on cell-cycle progression of human gastric cancer cells. Department of Preventive Medicine, Kyoto Prefectural University of Medicine, Japan. (August

1997). *NCBI PubMed.* Retrieved from https://www.ncbi.nlm.nih.gov/pubmed/8574744

Matthew Jenkin. Could mushrooms be the cure for cancer?. (March 3rd 2014). *The Guardian.* Retrieved from https://www.theguardian.com/lifeandstyle/2014/mar/02/could-mushrooms-cure-cancer

Mawson AR, Ray BD, Bhuiyan AR, Jacob B (2017) Pilot comparative study on the health of vaccinated and unvaccinated 6- to 12-year-old U.S. children. J Transl Sci 3: DOI: 10.15761/JTS.1000186. Retrieved from https://www.oatext.com/Pilot-comparative-study-on-the-health-of-vaccinated-and-unvaccinated-6-to-12-year-old-U-S-children.php#Article

Mayo Clinic Staff. Gene Therapy. (n.d). *Mayo Clinic.* Retrieved from https://www.mayoclinic.org/tests-procedures/gene-therapy/about/pac-20384619

Measles among vaccinated Quebec kids questioned The Canadian Press Posted. (Oct 20, 2011). *Vaccine truth.* Retrieved from https://vaccinetruth.org/vaccines-dont-work.html

Melanoma facts and statistics. (n.d). *Melanoma Institute Australia.* Retrieved from https://www.melanoma.org.au/understanding-melanoma/melanoma-facts-and-statistics/

Melanoma Stats, Facts, and Figures. (n.d). *Aim at Melanoma Foundation.* Retrieved from https://www.aimatmelanoma.org/about-melanoma/melanoma-stats-facts-and-figures/

Melphalan. What Melphalan Is Used For. (n.d). *Chemocare.* Retrieved from http://chemocare.com/chemotherapy/drug-info/Melphalan.aspx

Michael Greger M.D. FACLM. Which Nut Fights Cancer Better?. (July 18th, 2014). *NutritionFacts.org.* Retrieved from https://nutritionfacts.org/video/which-nut-fights-cancer-better/

Mike Adams the health ranger. Vaccine horrors: Medical mutilation of innocent children exposed in Graphic photos of "safe" vaccines gone horribly wrong. (February 19, 2015). *Natural News.* Retrieved from https://www.naturalnews.com/048691_vaccine_damaged_children_graphic_photos_medical_mutilation.html

MonsantoVideoRevolt. (July 21st 2013). *Top 10 GMO foods to avoid.* [Video file]. Retrieved from https://www.youtube.com/watch?v=-LAKFhDguuw

Moritz, Andreas. (2007). *The Amazing Liver and Gallbladder Flush.* Published by Ener-Chi-Art for the liver: Andreas Moritz

Most Amazing Top 10. (Jun 1, 2016). *Top 10 Most Common Types Of Cancers.* [Video File]. Retrieved from https://www.youtube.com/watch?v=DT1kg4vKARE

Myeashea Alexander. (September 5, 2014). *The Rockstar Anthropologist.* Retrieved from https://therockstaranthropologist.wordpress.com/2014/09/05/self-trepanation-drilling-a-hole-in-your-own-head-watch/

Nancy Appleton PhD & G.N. 144 Reasons Sugar Ruins Your Health. (2015). *Nancy Appleton Books Health Blog*. Retrieved from https://nancyappleton.com/141-reasons-sugar-ruins-your-health/

Natural Cures. (Oct 25, 2016). *9 Home Remedies for Natural Colon Cleansing.* [Video file]. Retrieved from https://www.youtube.com/watch?v=hC7JWW4Z14Y

Nicole Cutler, L.Ac, MTCM, Dipl. Ac. (NCCAOM). (n.d). *Liver Support.* Retrieved from https://www.liversupport.com/3-safe-ways-to-detox-your-liver/

Nikolas Symbas MD. September 11, 2019. *What your urine is trying to tell you.* Retrieved from https://georgiaurologist.com/posts/news/urine-color-chart/

Nutri Neat Staff. Selenium Benefits. (April 9th 2018). *Nutri Neat.* Retrieved from https://nutrineat.com/selenium-benefits

One Green Planet. 10 Fascinating Facts about Cow's Milk. (2014). *One Green Planet.* Retrieved from https://www.onegreenplanet.org/natural-health/vegan-health/10-fascinating-facts-about-cows-milk/

Ovadje, P., Ammar, S., Guerrero, J. A., Arnason, J. T., & Pandey, S. (). Dandelion root extract affects colorectal cancer proliferation and survival through the activation of multiple death signalling pathways. *Oncotarget, 7*(45), 73080–73100. doi:10.18632/oncotarget.11485

Overdose Death Rates. (January 2019). *National Institute of Health – National Institute of Drug Abuse.* Retrieved from https://www.drugabuse.gov/related-topics/trends-statistics/overdose-death-rates

Owen Pearson. The toxicity of clove oil. (August 14th, 2017). *Livestrong.com.* Retrieved from https://www.livestrong.com/article/178693-the-toxicity-of-clove-oil/

Paul Fassa. Harry Hoxsey's cancer cure and his long war against the medical establishment. (n.d). *Health Impact News.* Retrieved from https://healthimpactnews.com/2016/harry-hoxseys-cancer-cure-and-his-long-war-against-the-medical-establishment/

Patocka J. University of South Bohemia, Ceské Budejovice, Faculty of Health and Social Care, Department of Radiology and Toxicology, Czech Republic. Organic lead toxicology. (2008). *NCBI PubMed.* Retrieved from https://www.ncbi.nlm.nih.gov/pubmed/19453086

Patricia Phillips. Deadly cures? – Many Medications pack a potentially lethal dose of fluoride. (2001). *Rense.com.* Retrieved from https://rense.com/general12/fl.htm

Pavitra Sampath. 10 reasons smoking is bad for you. (May 31st 2017). *The health site.* Retrieved from https://www.thehealthsite.com/diseases-conditions/10-reasons-smoking-is-bad-for-you/

Plato Smith. (Oct 17, 2018). *Deadly Deception, Exposing the Dangers of Vaccines.* [Video file]. Retrieved from https://www.youtube.com/watch?v=X8CyVkgDKvo

Phi, L., Sari, I. N., Yang, Y. G., Lee, S. H., Jun, N., Kim, K. S., Kwon, H. Y. (2018). Cancer Stem Cells (CSCs) in Drug Resistance and their Therapeutic Implications in Cancer Treatment. *Stem cells international, 2018,* 5416923. doi:10.1155/2018/5416923

Poison Dart Frog Wikipedia – File. Ranitomeya amazonica.jpg Created: (21 October 2006) This image, which was originally posted to Picasa Web Albums, was reviewed on 20 January 2011 by
the administrator or reviewer Wikitanvir, who confirmed that it was available on Picasa Web Albums under the above license on that date. https://commons.wikimedia.org/wiki/File:Ranitomeya_amazonica.jpg

Pub Chem. Formaldehyde. (n.d). *US National Library of Medicine - National Center for Biotechnology Information.* Retrieved from https://pubchem.ncbi.nlm.nih.gov/compound/712

Professor Marjorie Cohn and Jonathan Moore. The Vietnam War is not history for victims of Agent Orange. (October 9th 2017). *Global Research Centre.* Retrieved from https://www.globalresearch.ca/the-vietnam-war-is-not-history-for-victims-of-agent-orange/5612535

Prostate Cancer – Patient Version. (n.d). *National Cancer Institute.* Retrieved from http://www.cancer.gov/types/prostate

Prostate cancer statistics. (Tue, 21/05/19). *Australian Government Cancer Australia.* Retrieved from https://prostate-cancer.canceraustralia.gov.au/statistics

Ptkfgs. Georgia Guidestones. (January 2, 2018). *Wikimedia Commons.* Retrieved from https://en.wikipedia.org/w/index.php?curid=41675095

Ralph W. Moss, Ph.D. How effective is chemotherapy. (n.d). *International centre for Nutritional research, Inc. (Since 1981).* Retrieved from http://www.icnr.com/articles/ischemotherapyeffective.html

Residential Formaldehyde Testing. (n.d). *Future Proof Property Inspections.* Retrieved from https://fppi.ca/residential-formaldehyde-testing/

Revolutionloveevolve. (Mar 15, 2013). *Rupert Sheldrake - The Science Delusion banned ted talk.* [Video file]. Retrieved from https://www.youtube.com/watch?v=JKHUaNAxsTg

Risto Hot Sir. Linus Pauling. (November 6th 2018). *Wikiquote.* Retrieved from https://en.wikiquote.org/w/index.php?title=Linus_Pauling&oldid=2498942

Robert Jackler. (n.d.). *More Doctors Smoke Camels Than Any Other Cigarette.* Stanford research. Retrieved from http://tobacco.stanford.edu/tobacco_main/images.php?

token2=fm_st001.php&token1=fm_img0002.php&theme_file=fm_mt001.php&theme_name=Doctors%20Smoking&subtheme_name=More%20Doctors%20Smoke%20Camels

Rothkranz, Markus. (2012). *Free Food and Medicine.* Retrieved from HealAnything.com

Rupal Parekh. Rewind – 1949 Cigarette spot declares 'doctors smoke camels. (August 13, 2012). *ADAGE.* Retrieved from https://adage.com/article/news/rewind-1949-cigarette-spot-declares-doctors-smoke-camels/236635

Sarah Knapton. Chemotherapy warning as hundreds die from cancer-fighting drugs. (August 30, 2016). *The Telegraph.* Retrieved from https://www.telegraph.co.uk/science/2016/08/30/chemotherapy-warning-as-hundreds-die-from-cancer-fighting-drugs/

Sarah Pope MGA. (May 15, 2019). *The Healthy Home Economist.* Retrieved from https://www.thehealthyhomeeconomist.com/detox-baths-which-ones-are-best-and-for-what-ailments/

Sayer Ji, Founder. (May 7th 2018). *Green Med Info.* Retrieved from http://www.greenmedinfo.com/blog/25-cancer-stem-cell-killing-foods-smarter-chemo-radiation

Sayer Ji, Founder. Gandhi's Anti-Vaccine Views Ring True A Century Later. (February 1st 2015). *Green Med Info.* Retrieved from http://www.greenmedinfo.com/blog/gandhis-anti-vaccine-views-ring-true-century-laterA

Scott Crawford. (Aug 7, 2013). *Starving Cancer Cells to Death.* [Video file]. Retrieved from https://www.youtube.com/watch?v=om2Uj07ypec

Science News for Students. Bethany Brookshire. (August 26, 2019). *The pH scale.* Retrieved from https://www.sciencenewsforstudents.org/article/scientists-say-ph

Shalailah Medhora. Pharmaceuticals officially more of an issue than illicit drugs. (December 19, 2017). *Triple J Hack.* Retrieved from https://www.abc.net.au/triplej/programs/hack/misuse-of-pharmaceuticals-on-the-rise/9271046

Shawn Stevenson. Health Benefits Of Brazil Nuts – The Anti-Cancer Superfood. (n.d). *The Model Health Show.* Retrieved from https://themodelhealthshow.com/benefits-of-brazil-nuts/

Shebaby, W. N., Mroueh, M., Bodman-Smith, K., Mansour, A., Taleb, R. I., Daher, C. F., & El-Sibai, M. (2014). Daucus carota pentane-based fractions arrest the cell cycle and increase apoptosis in MDA-MB-231 breast cancer cells. *BMC complementary and alternative medicine, 14,* 387. doi:10.1186/1472-6882-14-387

Sherri Griffin. Drinking dirt: Bentonite clay detox. (February 2nd 2014). *Overthrow Martha.* Retrieved from http://www.overthrowmartha.com/2014/02/drinking-dirt-bentonite-clay-detox.html

Shiwani, S., Singh, N. K., & Wang, M. H. (2012). Carbohydrase inhibition and anti-cancerous and free radical scavenging properties along with DNA and protein protection ability of methanolic root extracts of Rumex crispus. *Nutrition research and practice, 6*(5), 389–395. doi:10.4162/nrp.2012.6.5.389

Singh, G. K., Yadav, V., Singh, P., & Bhowmik, K. T. (2017). Radiation-Induced Malignancies Making Radiotherapy a "Two-Edged Sword": A Review of Literature. *World journal of oncology, 8*(1), 1–6. doi:10.14740/wjon996w

Singh, Y., & Bali, C. (2013). Cannabis extract treatment for terminal acute lymphoblastic leukemia with a Philadelphia chromosome mutation. *Case reports in oncology, 6*(3), 585–592. doi:10.1159/000356446

Skin Cancer (Including Melanoma) – Patient Version. (March 15th 2018). *National Cancer Institute.* Retrieved from https://www.cancer.gov/types/skin

Skippy hereitcomesskippy. (Mar 28, 2017). *How I solved the Georgia guide stones.* [Video file]. Retrieved from https://www.youtube.com/watch?v=zQbXvb0EaUM

Sparks & Honey Cultural Strategists. (22 May, 2013) *Big think.* Retrieved from https://bigthink.com/amped/humans-10-human-and-90-bacterial

Spinelli, J. B, Yoon, H., Ringel, A. E., Jeanfavre, S, Clish, C. B., & Haigis, M. C. Metabolic recycling of ammonia via glutamate dehydrogenase supports breast cancer biomass. *Science (New York, N.Y.), 358*(6365), 941–946.

doi:10.1126/science.aam9305. (November 17). *NCBI PubMed.* Retrieved from https://www.ncbi.nlm.nih.gov/pubmed/29025995

Stephanie Seneff. Information on Glyphosate (Roundup). (n.d). *Stephanie Seneff.* Retrieved from https://people.csail.mit.edu/seneff/

Steven Nemeroff, ND. Preventing Surgery-Induced Cancer Metastasis. (December 2009). *Life extension.* Retrieved from https://www.lifeextension.com/magazine/2009/12/preventing-surgery-induced-cancer-metastasis/page-01

Stewart Cowan's Blog. A Poison on Most People's Shopping Lists. (September 9th 2013). *Real Street.* Retrieved from https://www.realstreet.co.uk/2013/09/a-poison-on-most-peoples-shopping-lists

Study indicates Opiates already in body may encourage cancer growth, certain medications could slow it. (December 12, 2012). *American Society of Anesthiologists.* Retrieved from https://www.asahq.org/about-asa/newsroom/news-releases/2012/12/study-indicates-opiates-already-in-body-may-encourage-cancer-growth

Study: Sugar hidden in junk food eight times more addictive than cocaine. (February 25th 2015). *ABC 13 Eye witness news.* Retrieved from https://abc13.com/health/study-sugar-is-as-addictive-as-cocaine/533979/

Taylor, W. F., & Jabbarzadeh, E. (2017). The use of natural products to target cancer stem cells. *American journal of cancer research, 7*(7), 1588–1605.

TB Rates in the United States 1982-2017. (March 22, 2018). *U.S. Centres for Disease Control and Prevention.* Retrieved from https://www.cdc.gov/nchhstp/newsroom/multimedia-resources/tb-multimedia-resources.html

TED-Ed. (Jan 7, 2014). *How sugar affects the brain.* [Video file]. Retrieved from https://www.youtube.com/watch?v=lEXBxijQREo

TED. (Aug 12, 2013). *Margaret Heffernan: The dangers of "willful blindness".* [Video file]. Retrieved https://www.youtube.com/watch?v=Kn5JRgz3W0o

Ted X Talks. (Apr 15, 2016). *Starving cancer away | Sophia Lunt | Tedxmsu.* [Video file]. Retrieved from https://www.youtube.com/watch?v=f6rSuJ2YheQ

The Carcinogenic Potency Project - Ammonium Hydroxide. (October 3, 2007). *Berkeley lab, the University of California.* Retrieved from https://toxnet.nlm.nih.gov/cpdb/chempages/AMMONIUM%20HYDROXIDE.html

The Dean. (Jul 14, 2013). *The Cancer Conspiracy.* [Video File]. Retrieved from https://www.youtube.com/watch?v=Tx7W662gd8M

The Progressive Radio Network. (Oct 23, 2015). *Death by Medicine a film by Gary Null.* [Video file]. Retrieved from https://www.youtube.com/watch?v=RwCUDCQMLwY

The Progressive Radio Network. (May 23, 2013). *Seeds of Death: Unveiling The Lies of GMO's - Full Movie.* [Video file]. Retrieved from https://www.youtube.com/watch?v=a6OxbpLwEjQ

The Stem Cell Theory of Cancer. (2018). *Stanford Medicine/Ludwig Centre.* Retrieved from http://med.stanford.edu/ludwigcenter/overview/theory.html

The Watchman. (Nov 25, 2016). *Genetic Roulette The Gamble of Our Lives.* [Video file]. Retrieved from https://www.youtube.com/watch?v=7sUNxX0OxP8

Think Tank. (Nov 3, 2015). *8 Terrifying Effects Sugar Has On Your Body.* [Video file]. Retrieved from https://www.youtube.com/watch?v=_mBoI-F4K4o

This is Whats Going On. (Aug 19, 2015). *Silent Epidemic - The untold story of vaccines.* [Video file]. Retrieved from https://www.youtube.com/watch?v=mTjvX6s2Jvk

Thrive Movement. (Apr 5, 2012). *(Official Movie) Thrive: What On Earth Will It Take?.* [Video file]. Retrieved from https://www.youtube.com/watch?v=lEV5AFFcZ-s

Tkarcher. Vaccines Herd Immunity. (March 3, 2017). *Wikimedia Commons.* Retrieved from https://commons.wikimedia.org/w/index.php?curid=56760604

Tohme, S., Simmons, R. L., & Tsung, A. (2017). Surgery for Cancer: A Trigger for Metastases. *Cancer research, 77*(7), 1548–1552. doi:10.1158/0008-5472.CAN-16-1536

Toxic Substances Portal - Ammonia. (September 2004). *Agency for toxic Substances & Disease Registry.* Retrieved from https://www.atsdr.cdc.gov/PHS/PHS.asp?id=9&tid=2

Tracie White. Most physicians would forgo aggressive treatment for themselves at the end of life, study finds. (May 28, 2014). *Stanford Medicine News Center.* Retrieved from https://med.stanford.edu/news/all-news/2014/05/most-physicians-would-forgo-aggressive-treatment-for-themselves-.html

Trepanation on Wikipedia – Trepanated skull of a woman-Tumb 3 Corseaux-En Seyton-on display 6. Origional work by RAMA 14:19, 24 September 2006. Retrieved from https://commons.wikimedia.org/wiki/File:Trepanated_skull_of_a_woman-P4140363-black.jpg

Truly Heal. (Nov 17, 2016). *Cancer is curable now (Original Documentary).* [Video file]. Retrieved from https://www.youtube.com/watch?v=0R7K3OhaYLs

Ty Bollinger. 5 Medicinal Mushrooms That Fight Cancer. (March 19th, 2019). *The Truth about Cancer.* Retrieved from https://thetruthaboutcancer.com/medicinal-mushrooms-cancer/

UAMS Winthrop P. Rockefeller Cancer Institute. Radiation Therapy Facts. (n.d). *UAMS health.* Retrieval from https://uamshealth.com/medicalservices/cancer/cancer treatments/radiationfacts/

Ulrich Arndt. Salvestrols - A New Therapy against Cancer. (n.d). *Horus Media.* Retrieved from http://www.horusmedia.de/2010-salvestrole/salvestrole-en.php

Understand the issues. 35 FDA-Approved Prescription Drugs Later Pulled from the Market. (January 30th 2014). *Procon.org.* Retrieved from http://prescriptiondrugs.procon.org/view.resource.php?resourceID=005528

Urine Color Chart. (n.d). *Healthinfocu.net.* Retrieved from http://www.herbs-info.com/blog/wp-content/uploads/2015/05/Urine-Color-Chart.gif

Vaccine Ingredients and Manufacturer Information: Alphabetical order by vaccine. (September 19th 2016). *Procon.com.* Retrieved from https://vaccines.procon.org/view.resource.php?resource ID=005206#influenza

Watchdog USA. (n.d). *Death by Vaccination.* Retrieved from http://deathbyvaccination.com/

What can I do with Ammonia. (n.d). *Ammonia – NH3.* Retrieved from https://ammonianh3.weebly.com/what-can-i-do-with-ammonia.html

What is cancer. (February 9, 2015). *National Cancer Institute.* Retrieved from http://www.cancer.gov/about-cancer/understanding/what-is-cancer#types-of-cancer

What's In a Cigarette. (n.d). American Lung Association. Retrieved from https://www.lung.org/stop-smoking/smoking-facts/whats-in-a-cigarette.html

What Sugar Does to Your Brain. (n.d). *Factual Facts.* Retrieved from https://factualfacts.com/sugar-brain/

William Brown. Scientists Show That Water Has Memory. (October 15, 2018). Resonance Science Foundation. Retrieved from https://resonance.is/scientists-show-that-water-has-memory/

Wolfe ND, Dunavan CP, Diamond J. Origins of Major Human Infectious Diseases. Institute of Medicine (US). Improving Food Safety Through a One Health Approach: Workshop Summary. Washington (DC): National Academies Press (US). (2012). *NCBI Bookshelf.* Retrieved from https://www.ncbi.nlm.nih.gov/books/NBK114494/

Worldwide Cancer Data – Global cancer statistics for the most common types of cancer. (2018). *World cancer research fund /American institute for cancer research.* Retrieved from https://www.wcrf.org/dietandcancer/cancer-trends/worldwide-cancer-data

Worldwide Cancer Statistics. (n.d). *Cancer research UK.* Retrieved from https://www.cancerresearchuk.org/health-professional/cancer-statistics/worldwide-cancer.

Wu L[1], Guo L[1], Liang Y[1], Liu X[1], Jiang L[1], Wang L[1]. School of Chemistry and Chemical Engineering, Guangxi University, Nanning, Guangxi. Curcumin suppresses stem-like traits of lung cancer cells via inhibiting the JAK2/STAT3 signalling pathway. (September 16th 2015). *NCBI PubMed.* Retrieved from http://www.ncbi.nlm.nih.gov/pubmed/26397387

Zachary Shahan. Monsanto & Federal Governments Revolving Ties. (n.d). *Planet Save.* Retrieved from https://planetsave.com/2012/02/03/monsanto-federal-governments-revolving-ties/

Zhang, B., Zhang, X., Li, M., Kong, L., Deng, X., & Yu, J. (). How breast cancer chemotherapy increases the risk of leukemia: Thoughts about a case of diffuse large B-cell lymphoma and leukemia after breast cancer chemotherapy. *Cancer biology & therapy, 17*(2), 125–128. doi:10.1080/15384047.2016.1139233

2,4-D. (2016). *PAN Pesticide Database – Chemicals.* Retrieved from http://www.pesticideinfo.org/Detail_Chemical.jsp?Rec_Id=PC33097

For any references that I may have forgotten or misspelt credit will be given where it is due along with my sincerest apologies... Thank you for all of your hard work!

Notes:

Notes:

Notes:

Notes:

Notes:

Notes:

Notes:

Notes:

Made in United States
North Haven, CT
21 August 2025

71962326R00226